Listening to Your Own Body

Listening to Your Own Body

A Guide to the Neurological Problems That Afflict Us as We Grow Older

JAMES W. NEUMANN, M.D.

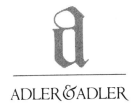

ADLER&ADLER

Published in the United States in 1987 by
Adler & Adler, Publishers, Inc.
4550 Montgomery Avenue
Bethesda, Maryland 20814

Library of Congress Cataloging-in-Publication Data
Neumann, James W., 1924
   Listening to your own body.
   1. Nervous system—Diseases—Age factors—Popular
works.   2. Nervous system—Diseases—Diagnosis—
Popular works.   3. Aged—Diseases—Diagnosis—Popular
works.   4. Self-examination, Medical.   I. Title.
[DNLM: 1. Nervous System Diseases—in old age—
popular works. WL 100 N489L]
RC351.N49 1986 618.97'68 86-7985
ISBN 0-917561-22-8
ISBN 0-917561-26-0 (Pbk.)

Printed in the United States of America

First Edition

To my wife, Ann

Contents

Acknowledgments   ix

Introduction   1

Symptom Index   5

1 Carpal Tunnel Syndrome   9

2 Bell's Palsy, Hemifacial Spasm,
   Restless Legs   13

3 Shingles   17

4 Syncope   21

5 Headache   25

6 Facial Pain   35

7 Peripheral Neuropathy   41

8 Tardive Dyskinesia   49

9 Myasthenia Gravis   53

10 Alcoholism   57

11 Seizures   63

12 Stroke   71

13 Parkinson's Disease   81

14 Alzheimer's Disease and Other
   Dementias   91

Contents

15 Amyotrophic Lateral Sclerosis   105

16 Drugs: Side Effects   109

Afterword   119

Glossary   121

Acknowledgments

to Bill Dickinson—for his help and encouragement
to Dewey K. Ziegler, M.D.—for his critique and advice

Introduction

PERHAPS you're wondering, "What's so unique about this book?"

The answer is that your body is constantly sending you signals about the state of your health. Some of these signals are simply symptoms of age, but others are symptoms of disease. This book will help you distinguish between the two.

When I began practicing medicine some thirty years ago, symptoms reported by patients were a central part of the diagnostic process. But as medical technology has improved, doctors have become more and more dependent upon laboratory tests. Attention to your symptoms doesn't seem quite as important as it used to be.

But there is a family of diseases—the neurological ailments—for which there are no definitive laboratory tests. Would you believe there are no specific tests that tell the physician his patient has Parkinson's disease, tic douloureux, essential tremor, meralgia paresthetica, Alzheimer's disease, or migraines? This is an imposing list, but one that is far from complete.

Neurological diseases like these particularly attack as we grow older. Each year, countless people over sixty contract these ailments, and not all of them have easy access to a neurologist—there are about eight thousand of us in the United States.

So if you're in the target age group, you and your general practitioner or internist must listen to your symptoms very carefully to determine whether you have a neurological disease.

Here is how to use *Listening to Your Own Body*:

1. If you have a specific symptom that bothers you —for instance, you're having some difficulty swallowing—first look it up in the Symptom Index. You'll find references to the pages that describe the different diseases or group of related ailments in which patients generally experience difficulty swallowing.

2. Compare your symptoms with the overall disease descriptions in these pages. For example, pages 18 and 35–39 refer to three different ailments that cause facial pain; pages 53–56 deal with myasthenia gravis, a "block" in the transmission of the nerve impulses that often causes weakness in the pharynx or swallowing mechanism; pages 105–108 discuss amyotrophic lateral sclerosis, or Lou Gehrig's disease, an ailment that affects motor nerve cells and causes increasing weakness in arms, legs, facial muscles and the swallowing mechanism.

3. On these pages you will also be told how serious each disease is and, generally speaking, what the most common treatments are. You will be warned about the possible side effects of medication that may be prescribed. In addition, a checklist that sums up the symptoms of each disease follows each

chapter in order to make it easier for you to communicate with your doctor.

4. If you find that one of these detailed descriptions seems to match the signals you're getting from your body, it's probably time for you to discuss the matter with your doctor.

It's not my purpose to suggest that this book is a substitute for sound medical advice from your own doctor, or to make people over sixty into amateur neurologists. It *is* my intent to make you better informed about your symptoms, and better able to help your physician make a diagnosis.

Remember, the earlier your doctor makes a correct diagnosis, the greater your chances for prompt treatment and effective relief. Help *him* help *you.* That's what this book is all about.

Symptom Index

THIS index provides you with a quick reference to the page or pages where a particular symptom is discussed. Pain, weakness, numbness and difficulty walking are common to many neurological disorders, so reference to many pages has been necessary.

Designation by body parts simplifies the use of the index. See the Glossary for the definition of a term that may be unfamiliar to you.

Symptom

amnesia, 75

blackouts, 59

consciousness, loss of, 21, 30

convulsions, 63–70

dizziness, 109, 114–117

eye problems

    double vision, 55, 59, 73

    droopy eyelid, 53

    eye closure, 50

    field of vision limited, 28, 72

facial immobility (lack of expression), 52, 74

Symptom

  paralysis, 13

fainting, 21, 116

hallucinations, 59, 113

headache, 25–34

impotence, 59

insomnia, 16

memory loss, 59, 91

movement

  involuntary, 50, 65, 66, 67, 112

  slow, 82

numbness

  arm, 44, 59, 64, 73

  face, 64, 74

  fingertips, 42, 97

  foot, 43, 59, 97

  hand, 9, 42, 44, 74, 97

  leg, 41, 61, 64, 73

  lip, 74

  trunk, 74

pain

  arm, 44, 59

  face, 18, 35–39

Symptom

   head, 18, 25–34

   leg, 41, 59

   neck, 38

   throat, 38

   trunk, 17

   shoulder, 85

   wrist, 9–12

rigidity (stiffness), 82, 85

seizures, 60, 63–70

speaking difficulties, 61, 75

swallowing difficulties (*see also* weakness,
   swallowing), 38, 53, 106

taste, loss of, 13

tearing, 13, 29

tingling sensation

   hand, 9, 44, 97

   leg, 41, 64, 97

tremor, 61, 81, 82–84

twitching

   eye, 14

   face, 14, 65

   hand, 65

   leg, 14, 64

Symptom

walking difficulties, 42, 59, 61, 74, 84, 106

weakness

    arm, 44, 53, 61, 74, 105

    face, 14, 74

    hand, 9, 59

    leg, 17, 43, 45, 53, 59, 61, 73, 105

    respiration, 45, 55

    swallowing, 54

1. Carpal Tunnel Syndrome

MAJOR problems like Parkinson's disease, stroke and dementia deserve serious consideration; so what about a painful wrist? This doesn't sound serious, but it can be disabling. An eighty-year-old woman told me that she could not teach her aquatic aerobics class because of wrist pain. A seventy-year-old man was abandoning his woodworking shop. A sixty-eight-year-old woman could no longer knit and crochet because of the pain. A sixty-four-year-old man "retired" his tennis racquet. These may not seem to be earthshaking events, but they are certainly important to the people involved.

"Painful wrist" is actually carpal tunnel syndrome, which for some unknown reason affects more women than men.

The carpal tunnel lies deep in the wrist area. Through this structure pass tendons, blood vessels and nerves. One of these nerves is the median nerve. Compression of this nerve produces pain in the wrist and tingling in the fingers, primarily in the thumb, index and middle finger. Physicians differ in their treatment of carpal tunnel syndrome. Some will inject the wrist with a cortisone preparation and others will use a splint to immobilize and protect the wrist. In my experience, these measures afford temporary relief. A relatively simple surgical procedure, called a carpal tunnel release, is about 90 percent effective in relieving the symptoms. This procedure is usually performed on an outpatient basis and involves relieving the pressure from the median nerve.

For years, wrist and hand pain was often attributed to arthritis. In many patients that is the problem, but in others it isn't necessarily the case. Arthritis is a common complaint in the aging population, and carpal tunnel syndrome often occurs in conjunction with existing arthritis.

The pain from carpal tunnel syndrome differs from arthritic pain, however, which should alert you to a new problem. The symptoms usually begin as an aching discomfort in the wrist, thumb and index finger. Frequently people complain of the entire hand hurting. Activities such as writing, holding the telephone, holding a newspaper, opening a jar, combing hair and driving the car will, after a few minutes, produce discomfort. One symptom that virtually all patients have is nocturnal pain. A patient will awaken with discomfort, get up, walk about, shake his arm and go back to bed, only to get up again because the pain recurs. A small number of patients will complain of forearm pain in addition to pain in the wrist and hand.

Most people will seek medical attention shortly after the onset of symptoms. At the age of sixty-five or older the probability of arthritis being diagnosed is high. "But Doc, I've never had arthritis before!" "Has to start some time—you're getting older, you know." Aspirin or an arthritis medication will probably be prescribed. The symptoms of carpal tunnel syndrome will *not* improve with medications. I would estimate that 80 percent of the patients I have seen over the age of sixty-five with carpal tunnel syndrome have been on arthritis medication. If you're convinced that you have arthritis, you may "just decide to live with it." As time passes, the thumb becomes weak because of muscle wasting due to nerve damage. This weakness causes difficulty in performing tasks such as turning a key, buttoning, writing and other acts that require fine motor control.

If a diagnosis of arthritis has been made and medications have not relieved your symptoms, what are you to do? Ask your doctor about the possibility of carpal tunnel syndrome. Fortunately, there is a simple nerve conduction study that, in most cases, proves the diagnosis. The study can be performed in the neurologist's office or at a hospital on an outpatient basis. A weak electric current stimulates the nerve at the wrist and then the upper arm; this procedure stings, but it is not painful. The study itself takes about twenty minutes and the results are known in one hour. I have mentioned that outpatient surgery is readily available and in most cases is performed with gratifying results.

The carpal tunnel syndrome is correctable. Early diagnosis is important for relief of pain and restoration of function. "Painful wrist": you know what to ask about, now.

CHECKLIST

READ the following for symptoms associated with carpal tunnel syndrome. Remember that nocturnal pain is almost always associated with this condition.

1. Pain in the wrist, hand and forearm that has not responded to medications for arthritis.

2. Pain in the wrist and hand associated with the following activities:
    a. writing
    b. holding a newspaper
    c. driving a car
    d. opening a jar
    e. typing
    f. combing hair
    g. using a tool such as a screw driver.

3. Any activity that involves cocking the wrist even slightly, will, after a few minutes, produce tingling and pain.

2. Bell's Palsy, Hemifacial Spasm, Restless Legs

Bell's Palsy

BELL's palsy may occur in any age group; however, when it occurs in the aging population, the first impression is—trouble! Going about your early morning activities one day you smile at yourself in the mirror and to your shock and surprise realize that one side of your face doesn't move. The first thought that occurs is: "I've had a stroke"! You drink some coffee and part of it runs down your chin. Food may not taste right, because on occasion the sense of taste may be impaired on one side of your tongue. The eye on the paralyzed side feels irritated because tears run onto your face rather than bathing the eye. Occasionally, sounds seem too loud in the ear on the affected side: a small muscle in the hearing "bones" may be paralyzed. Do you remember whether six or seven days ago your ear ached or if there was pain behind the ear? What has happened? The nerve to the facial muscles has been compressed in the bony canal that lies just behind the ear. Apart from these facial symptoms, you are your normal self. You should see your physician for confirmation that you have Bell's palsy and that you have not suffered a stroke. In about 80 percent of patients with Bell's palsy the symptoms clear within six to nine weeks. In a small percentage of patients the facial weakness does not clear, and in the remaining percentage partial recovery occurs. Although cortisone has been used in the treatment of Bell's palsy, many physicians feel that the probability of spontaneous recovery negates its use.

Hemifacial Spasm

Your eye twitches, as it has done before. This time, however, it hasn't stopped—after several days. After several weeks the upper portion of your face begins to twitch. You see your physician and the diagnosis of a tic or nervous habit is suggested. After a few months the entire side of your face is in constant motion. Your condition is diagnosed as hemifacial spasm. It is extremely unpleasant, and fortunately this facial spasm is relatively unusual. In many cases the reason for this condition is similar to the cause of tic douloureux (see chapter 6). Neurosurgical procedures may relieve or improve the spasm. One operative series provides 60 to 70 percent relief. Complications associated with the procedure should be discussed with your physician. You may prefer to be operated on with the chance of improvement than put up with the spasm.

Restless Legs

"Doc, after thirty years of marriage we're not sleeping together."
"Sounds like a domestic problem."

"No, I can't stand his thrashing about in the bed!"

This is a common complaint in a case of restless legs syndrome. It's unusual to see this problem in anyone under the age of sixty. The symptoms of restless legs appear at bedtime. A variety of symptoms may be reported, such as crawling, itching, burning and wormlike movements under the skin, among others. These sensations are commonly associated with irresistable movements of the legs, which may help to quell or stop the feeling. Frequently you must get up and walk about to obtain relief. After you return to bed, the symptoms tend to recur. This syndrome may occur in cases of chronic kidney failure, but often it occurs for no apparent reason. Some drugs induce a condition called akathisia, which resembles the restless legs syndrome. Leg movements with akathisia occur during the day, whereas restless legs syndrome occurs predominantly at night.

This condition really doesn't sound serious, but after weeks of sleep-interrupted nights, it is. When you describe your symptoms to your physician, mention restless legs. In many cases the restless legs syndrome has responded to the medication Clonopin. Relief should occur in the first week, and a low maintenance dosage should keep the symptoms in check.

CHECKLIST

THE following will identify symptoms that you may not have noticed early in the development of the conditions discussed, so it may be necessary to recall symptoms that you experienced some time ago.

Bell's Palsy

1. Pain in or behind the ear

2. Food doesn't taste right

3. Usual sounds seem loud

4. Tears run down your face

5. One side of your face sags and is expressionless

Hemifacial Spasm

1. Eye twitches—may or may not be a problem

2. Eye and cheek twitch together

3. Twitch involves the entire side of the face

Restless Legs

1. Insomnia

2. Restlessness—need to get up and walk

3. Unpleasant or uncontrollable sensations in the leg

3. Shingles

SHINGLES is miserable to have. It occurs more often over the age of sixty and usually clears in eight to ten weeks, but occasionally pain can persist for months or up to a year or two. Shingles is caused by the virus herpes zoster, which is also the virus that causes chicken pox. Most people who develop shingles have had chicken pox in childhood.

Shingles usually develop over the back and chest wall, occasionally over the forehead and eye, and less often over the buttock and leg. When the buttock and leg are involved, weakness of the leg may be present. Itching, burning and/or pain in any of these sites is the earliest symptom. If you were to see your doctor within the first two or three days after the onset of symptoms, the diagnosis would be obscure. After the fourth or fifth day, blisterlike skin lesions appear in the areas affected with pain. At this time the diagnosis of shingles is apparent.

A bout of shingles is a painful experience. Treatment consists primarily of effecting relief from the pain, itching and burning. Cortisone or its derivatives may be used and may shorten the course of shingles. After the skin lesions have healed, usually in eight to ten weeks, small scars may remain on the skin. The sensation in the affected area may be dulled to the touch and remain so. The use of cortisone during the active phase of shingles also might prevent the pain following the initial bout.

Post-herpetic neuralgia, the pain that persists after the shingles attack, is distressing and most difficult to treat. Pain relief medications may be necessary for long periods of time. The use of cortisone during the active phase of shingles (six weeks) should not create significant side effects; however, cortisone should not be used for long-term treatment. Surgical procedures that have been used are sectioning or cutting the involved sensory nerve at its entry into the spinal cord or destroying the spinal tract that carries pain fibers. But none of these procedures has been highly successful. Many patients with post-herpetic neuralgia will recover in a year's time; others may be plagued with pain for years and require chronic pain relief.

If the shingles involve the upper face and eye, special attention must be given to the eye. Scarring of the cornea of the eye may occur, and vision could be impaired. Under these circumstances I feel that an ophthalmologist should be consulted and should follow the patient throughout the illness.

Why does shingles occur mostly in the aging population? We know that as we age we are, in general, physically slower than we once were. It takes the body longer to recover from operations, pneumonia and heart attacks. Our immune system, the system that directs the fight against infection, also works a little more slowly. It is presumed that this slower, less effective immune system allows the herpes zoster virus to proliferate and cause its damage.

Shingles, although painful and disagreeable, usually lasts for a relatively short time. If those of us who had chicken pox were to live long enough—say, to our eighties or nineties—we would be at high risk for a bout with shingles.

CHECKLIST

THE diagnosis of shingles almost always is made *after* the appearance of the skin lesions.

1. Have you had the recent onset of pain in your leg, arm or chest wall?

2. Have you checked for blisterlike lesions in the areas affected by pain four or five days after its onset?

3. Have your skin lesions healed and the pain persisted?

4. Syncope

ALMOST everyone as he grows older has fainted or has felt faint at some time. These events are termed "syncopal episodes" and have many different possible causes. Fainting entails the loss or near loss of consciousness, and in many cases is preceded by a feeling of light-headedness, nausea, sweating, weakness, blurred vision or ringing in the ears. Fainting usually occurs when you are standing and occasionally when you are in a sitting position.

An "understandable" faint occurs in some people when they hear terrible news, witness an accident or see blood. This is accepted as "one of those things" that can happen to people, and little is thought about it. If these stress-related fainting spells occur frequently, you should see your doctor and tell him about the circumstances that caused you to faint.

Then there's fainting of a more unusual nature. After arising in the morning, a man goes to the bathroom. He is standing at the commode urinating and the next thing he remembers is his wife asking, "What happened?" He is lying on the bathroom floor and he also wonders what happened. He has had an experience with "micturitional (act of urinating) syncope." This occurs only in males, and the cause is not known. This is a benign form of syncope and does not herald the onset of any disease.

Certainly, you might bang your head or otherwise injure yourself during the fall. My only suggestion is, sit to urinate.

Many people have a chronic cough due to bronchitis, emphysema or some other pulmonary disease. After a prolonged coughing spell, some people may faint and fall. The reason is presumed to be a slowing of the heart secondary to the protracted coughing. This kind of faint, brought on by a fit of coughing, is termed "tussive syncope." Tussive syncope can occur regularly in some people. You should see your doctor to be sure that no other cause might be responsible for your fainting.

You have been treated for high blood pressure (hypertension), and your doctor has recently made a change in your medication. You notice that when you get up after sitting for a period of time you feel unsteady, "faintlike," but within seconds you're fine. After standing in a line for ten minutes at a checkout counter, you look at your watch and wonder what the holdup is. The next thing you remember is lying on the floor with someone asking if you're all right. Fainting frequently occurs due to a drop in your blood pressure (hypotension) induced by some high blood pressure medications. Look for the simplest explanation of the faint—a recent change in medication. If you have hypertension, having a blood pressure cuff at home is a good way to monitor what the medication is doing. Have someone check your blood pressure when you are lying down and after you have been standing for a short period of time. You may find a considerable drop in blood pressure when standing, and this may be accompanied by faintlike symptoms. This is called "postural hypotension." If these circumstances exist, check with your doctor regarding medication management.

Two medications used in the management of Parkinson's disease can also cause postural hypotension. They are Sinemet and Parlodel. Your symptoms of Parkinson's disease may improve rapidly soon after beginning the medication, but you may feel light-headed and dizzy at times. Tell your physician about the symptoms and mention the possibility of a drop in blood pressure. Medication adjustments can be made to control both the symptoms of Parkinson's disease and postural hypotension.

Fainting episodes may also be caused by heartbeat irregularities and heart disease. Some diabetics may have a complicating postural hypotension. If you are a diabetic or a heart patient, a fainting spell will suggest to your doctor a specific complication that may have occurred. In addition there are some unusual neurological disorders that result in postural hypotension and fainting.

Seizurelike activity may occur during the unconscious period of a faint. Under these conditions even the most skilled observer has difficulty in distinguishing faint-seizure from seizure alone. Your help in this situation is invaluable by relating, "I have fainted before and this time I remember feeling light-headed, sweaty and nauseated before I passed out."

Fainting from whatever cause carries with it the

risk of injury because of falling. An isolated fainting episode can probably be ignored, but repeated events need to be diagnosed and appropriate treatment for the problem initiated.

CHECKLIST

THE following questions will help you identify the cause of fainting.

1. When did you first faint?

2. How many times have you fainted?

3. Under what circumstances did the faint occur?

4. Did you notice an irregular heartbeat prior to the faint?

5. Are you being treated for heart disease?

6. Have you recently changed medications?

7. Do you have Parkinson's disease, hypertension or diabetes? Check with your doctor about medications.

5. Headache

Woe to the patient who has had headaches for thirty years. Woe to the physician whose patient has had headaches for thirty years. After writing ten different prescriptions, without relieving the patient's headache, the physician begins to feel miserable also. Headaches have always plagued mankind. They occur in all age groups, and in spite of new and innovative medications, they remain difficult to treat. There are many different causes for headaches: sinus infections, visual problems, ear infections—the list is endless. We will be concerned only with the neurological causes of headache. Obviously, an accurate description of your headaches enhances the probabilities of a correct diagnosis and appropriate treatment.

"Doc, I have a headache."

"Where?"

"In my head."

That answer isn't good enough.

Temporal Arteritis

Temporal arteritis occurs mostly in the over-sixty age group. The headache is usually unilateral (one-sided) and involves the temple. The pain frequently radiates to the forehead and the eye of the affected side. Initially the headache stutters: here today, gone tomorrow. It soon becomes constant. The temporal area becomes sensitive and painful to the touch. It is possible that you may have had migraine headaches for some time. Indeed, if at this stage of temporal arteritis you visit your physician, a diagnosis of migraine or "nonspecific" head pain may be made. If you have had migraines, *you* will recognize the change in the headache pattern from the occasional attack of migraine to the constant pain of temporal arteritis. In addition to the headache, you may develop aching and pain in your shoulders and thigh muscles. This condition is called "polymyalgia rheumatica." You may develop temporary blindness on the side of the headache. In general, you feel fatigued and run down. You now have a full-blown case of temporal arteritis, and your vision could well be at stake. Now that you are aware of the progression of symptoms in temporal arteritis, you should know that an early diagnosis may well save you from potential visual loss and relieve the severe head pain.

Your detailed history should lead to confirming laboratory tests. A blood study, called the sedimentation rate, can be done. If the sedimentation rate is elevated, suggesting the possibility of temporal arteritis, the temporal artery is biopsied to confirm inflammatory changes in the artery. The pain of temporal arteritis is caused by an inflammatory change in the vessel wall. The reason for this change is unknown. It is not due to an infection. Treatment with Prednisone, a cortisone derivative, produces dramatic results. The temporal pain disappears and visual impairment is corrected. The Prednisone dosage is slowly decreased over six months to one year, and a small maintenance dose may be necessary thereafter. Remember, recognizing and describing to your doctor the progression of your symptoms remains the key to diagnosis.

Migraine Headache

People who suffer from migraine headaches usually get them before the age of sixty; however, the headaches frequently continue into the sixties. The headaches are unilateral (one-sided), and they occur in a paroxysmal pattern that differs for each individual, which means the headache may occur once a week, once a month or every three or six months. The pattern tends to remain the same for each individual. The tendency to develop migraine headaches occurs in 40 to 60 percent of the offspring of people with migraine. The genetic predisposition accounts for the largest number of patients with migraine.

Years ago migraine headaches were called "sick" headaches, and they still are "sick" headaches. They may occur on the right or left side, and the pain in many instances seems to be behind the eye. The headache is deep, throbbing and severe. Bright light tends to increase the severity of the headache and nausea and/or vomiting are usually present. Most patients seek a quiet, dark room to endure their misery. Once the headache has begun, medications are not of much value.

A unique feature of migraine headaches is the occurrence of symptoms prior to the onset of the headache. One of two things may happen. For a day or two prior to the onset of headache, you may feel irritable, fatigued and depressed. Then the headache sets up housekeeping. The second series of symptoms is much different and definitely more alarming than your first experience. Thirty to forty-five minutes prior to the onset of the headache, you could experience any of the following: temporary loss of vision, in the right or left visual field; bright lights exploding like a Roman candle; the illusion of lights flashing through a moving picket fence; numbness of the hands and/or face; numbness of half the body. Other events might occur, but those mentioned are most common. Stress, whether physical or emotional, may precipitate migraine headaches and migraine headaches may be precipitated by certain food products, such as cheese, or the chemicals in some canned soups. It's the physician's responsibility to advise the patient about this possibility, and it is your responsibility to relate the events that precede your migraines to your physician. It is possible, as one ages, for the headaches to disappear; however, the symptoms that preceded the headache may continue to occur.

Medications are available for the treatment of migraine headaches and are successful in a significant percentage of people affected. At the present time the most effective medication seems to be Propranolol. This is a prescription drug that may serve to prevent the occurrence of a migraine attack. If the headaches are infrequent, occurring every three to six months, ergot medication, such as Gynergan may be prescribed.

Cluster Headaches

Cluster headaches are so called because they occur in cycles or in clusters. They occur mostly in the under-fifty age group. I mention these headaches because they may become chronic and occur daily. Chronic cluster headaches extend into the over-sixty population. As in migraine, cluster headaches also occur on only one side of the head. The pain lies in or behind the eye, temple or face and is severe. The nose feels stuffy and the eye may water excessively. The headache may last forty-five minutes to one hour, only to recur later that day. The headaches frequently occur at night, and nobody sleeps through a cluster headache. Medications are available for the management of cluster and chronic cluster headaches. These headaches are difficult to treat, but successful management is possible with medication.

Subarachnoid Hemorrhage

A headache caused by subarachnoid hemorrhage is bad news, and I mention it only because prompt recognition and attention could be life saving. The headache usually is secondary to a *ruptured* aneurysm, the aneurysm being a balloonlike sac on a blood vessel. The headache occurs suddenly; one minute you're fine, the next minute you have the worst headache possible. The headache may occur with lifting and straining, or it may occur without any provocation. Consciousness may or may not be lost. The signal to this problem is an abrupt, sudden onset of severe headache that is devastating. It is essential to get to an emergency room as soon as possible. This is a *neurosurgical emergency;* prompt recognition and early treatment could save a life.

Muscle Tension Headaches

Muscle tension headaches, muscle contraction headaches, tension headaches, stress-related headaches—all form a part of the same headache constellation. These are the realm of the patient with headaches for thirty years and the realm of a frustrated physician. People with headaches over such a long period have invariably seen several physicians and have tried a variety of medications, none of which has been successful. These headaches are the kinds of headaches most people have—not migraine, cluster, sinus infections, etc.

Muscle tension headaches may begin in any portion of the head or neck. Frequently they begin in the neck and involve the back of the head. The neck muscles become tense, hence the term "muscle tension." The pain is described as a pressure sensation or a bandlike sensation around the head, like a tight-fitting hat. These headaches may last for days, weeks or months.

What are the causes of muscle tension headaches?

Every conceivable anxiety that people have or think they have. It would be futile to attempt an all-encompassing identification. Briefly, some stress-related situations that could cause a muscle tension headache are concern about the illness of a spouse, worry over getting older, worrying about money, or the mortgage, or Social Security, or a wayward child . . . the list is endless.

The reason why muscle tension headaches are so difficult to manage should be apparent. If the patient can't identify what's bothering him as the underlying cause of the headache, how can it be treated? I'm not sure how many over-the-counter and prescription drugs are available for the treatment of headaches, but new products with new names and wonderful claims and promises for relief are being introduced all the time. I am sure they will be purchased and tried without any more success than all the previous medications the patient has used.

Many patients with muscle tension headaches are concerned about the possibility of having a brain tumor. A CAT scan will prove the existence or the nonexistence of the tumor. The absence of a tumor should drop the anxiety level in those patients, thus alleviating their suffering. If only *all* the problem-causing headaches could be solved as simply as that!

A final word about muscle tension headaches: the clue to the cure lies with you. Headache medications can be of value, but it is more important for you to try to identify the problem. Then you must change the situation, if possible, or at least try to lower your level of anxiety. If it is not possible to modify the situation, and this is the hardest part, then you should learn to live with it. Counseling with your physician can be beneficial, but, unfortunately, most physicians will not take the time to become involved. Psychiatrists and other professional counselors are of value in helping to sort out and understand problems. Counseling services are not available in many areas of the country, so this method of treatment may not be possible. Learning to live with headache pain may not be pleasant, but often it is necessary.

There remains a significant number of patients who have headaches for no apparent cause. We hope within the next few years to have better definition and management of this troublesome symptom so that these people also can be helped.

In summary, there are no diagnostic tests that will identify migraine or cluster headaches, only your detailed description of your symptoms. Tests to confirm temporal arteritis will be ordered only after you relate your symptoms to your physician. Subarachnoid hemorrhage need not be fatal with *prompt* recognition and action. It is apparent that communication with your physician is vital to diagnosis in these situations.

CHECKLIST

HEADACHES are diagnosed by considering the following:

1. Location—"Where does it hurt?"
   a. temple
   b. whole head
   c. back of head
   d. front of head
   e. back of eye
   f. one-half of head

2. Duration since onset
   a. years
   b. months
   c. weeks
   d. hours

3. Duration of headache
   a. constant
   b. two days
   c. twenty-four hours
   d. one hour

4. Associated symptoms
   a. visual loss
   b. flashing lights
   c. blurred vision
   d. nausea/vomiting
   e. tearing of eye
   f. nasal stuffiness

    g. "band" around head

    h. neck pain

5. Precipitating causes

    a. alcohol

    b. cheese, canned soup

    c. "Three hours after I take that medicine"

    d. tension

6. Facial Pain

You talk and it hits you, you eat and it hits you, the wind blows on your face and it hits you: is it a tooth, a tic or what?

Tic Douloureux (Trigeminal Neuralgia)

The pain of tic douloureux is terrible; there are lots of other words for it. The quality of this pain has been described to me in a variety of ways: "It feels like a hot poker in my jaw"; "As if lightning struck me"; "Like a strong electrical shock"; "It feels just terrible—it's the worst pain I've ever had." I have seen patients who, when the pain strikes, grab their jaw, lean forward and cry.

The pain is located in either the lower or upper jaw on one side of the face, often involving the lower or upper teeth. Eating or talking will often precipitate an attack. During an attack of tic douloureux the following sequence will occur: the pain will strike, last thirty to forty-five seconds, let up for two or three minutes, then strike again. This could occur for several hours. The jaw, after several paroxysms of pain, becomes tender and sensitive. The characteristic pain recurs again and again.

I have seen several patients with tic douloureux who initially saw their dentist; the results of those visits were tooth extraction and, on occasion, root canal surgery. If your complaint is, "Doc, I've got this bad pain in my jaw," the appropriate response would be, "Where is it?"

"In my jaw."

"Do you think it's a tooth?"

"I don't know."

"See your dentist."

Let's take this a bit further: "Is the pain constant?"

"Pretty much so, but it gets worse at times."

"Is it tender here?"

"A little."

Sinus X-rays have been ordered and turn out normal. Where do we go from here? "See your dentist." This narrative, sad as it is, could be repeated many times. The assumption that if the pain is located in the jaw it must be a tooth isn't correct. Granted, there can be difficulty in separating tooth pain (usually constant, throbbing, aching and localized) from tic pain (stabbing, brief in duration with moments of relief between paroxysms), but there shouldn't be.

There does not appear to be a single common cause for tic douloureux, although some form of irritation occurs at the origin of the fifth cranial nerve (trigeminal nerve) or through its course from the brain to the face. During the past few years one cause has been identified. As we age, our blood vessels become more rigid. The blood vessels in the brain stem, where the trigeminal nerve emerges, lie in close proximity to the nerves. Pliable, pulsating vessels glide over the nerves, which do not compress them. Stiff, rigid vessels compress the nerves and irritability occurs. This cause of tic douloureux has been demonstrated many, many times by the neurosurgeon, when the vessel is successfully shifted and the pain is relieved. If, at the time of surgery, nerve compression is not found, other neurosurgical techniques are available. The neurosurgeon may elect to: inject the nerve with alcohol, section or cut the nerve, or electrocoagulate the nerve. But operations for tic douloureux are necessary *only* if medication fails to control the symptoms or when prolonged use of medication is required.

The first and subsequent attacks of tic douloureux usually respond to the medications Tegretol and/or Dilantin. Over a period of several weeks to a few months, medication needs to be continued. When you have been symptom-free—without pain —for several weeks, an attempt should be made to discontinue the medication by slowly lowering the dosage. You may then be pain-free without the medication and, if the pain recurs, medication may be resumed. You may remain pain-free for several months or years and then have another attack. Once again, the medication should control the symptoms. I repeat, neurosurgical procedures should be considered only when medications fail to control the symptoms or when prolonged use of medication is required.

Glossopharyngeal Neuralgia

The pain of glossopharyngeal neuralgia (pretty fancy words for pain in the throat and tonsillar areas) is similar in quality and characteristics to the pain of tic douloureux. The pain is precipitated by swallowing and, obviously, eating; therefore, maintaining an adequate diet becomes a problem. The condition is relatively rare, but it bears mentioning because the one person in a thousand who gets this might be you. Glossopharyngeal neuralgia is managed in the same manner as tic douloureux, and in many cases the cause for this neuralgia is the same. The description of your pain—location, duration, precipitating factors and type of pain—establishes the diagnosis.

Temporo-mandibular Joint Syndrome

If you place your finger in front of your ear, press in, then open your mouth, you will feel the temporo-mandibular joint. If your "bite" is off due to malocclusion or ill-fitting dentures, this joint becomes stressed, and pain will develop. The pain increases in severity when you chew. This pain can usually be well identified by its location and its aggravation by eating. Your dentist can help with this problem.

In summary, I cannot stress enough how important your specific history is in the diagnosis of facial pain and all other neurological problems.

CHECKLIST

THE following should help identify which of the three conditions, trigeminal neuralgia (TN), glossopharyngeal neuralgia (GN), or temporo-mandibular joint syndrome (TMJ), is responsible for your facial pain.

	TN	GN	TMJ
How long has the symptom been present?			
What is the character of the pain?	sharp stabbing	sharp stabbing	aching
How long does the pain last?	brief seconds	brief seconds	constant but fluctuates
Location of pain	lower jaw upper jaw	throat	upper jaw in front of ear
What aggravates the pain?	eating talking smiling touching jaw	eating swallowing	chewing

Although the pain of trigeminal neuralgia and glossopharyngeal neuralgia are similar, the location differentiates one from the other.

7. Peripheral Neuropathy

THIS term peripheral neuropathy, for our purposes, refers to sensory and motor (muscle) symptoms that are the result of a disease affecting the nerves going into the arms and legs. Sensory and motor symptoms will be discussed in the chapters dealing with strokes and seizures. Those symptoms are the result of a disease affecting the brain. The symptoms that arise from a peripheral neuropathy are due to involvement of the nerve itself, not the brain.

SENSORY

The most common complaint regarding sensory changes in the feet and legs is, "I think that my circulation is bad." Most people make this assumption because circulation problems to the heart and brain are more frequently found in the over-sixty population. Poor circulation can cause numbness and tingling in the extremities, but other reasons are found far more often.

The numbness, tingling, burning and other symptoms due to peripheral neuropathies are not transient features; they are constant. The numbness usually begins in the feet and slowly progresses up to the ankle and then to the midcalf. You may trip over objects more easily, stumble unexpectedly and have more difficulty placing your feet where they should be. At some time during the course of this progression, the fingertips may also become numb. Although the sensation of numbness is perceived only by the patient, outward signs may be apparent: dropping objects, inability to differentiate between coins, inability to pick up small objects, etc. The sensory symptoms of a peripheral neuropathy usually develop over weeks to months.

After a few weeks of symptoms, your first visit to the physician may be unrewarding. The doctor finds circulation is good in your legs and can detect no sensory loss in your feet, legs or hands. Here it comes: "You're getting older and you just don't feel things as well as you used to." Be persistent—on your next visit some blunting of sensation may be apparent to the physician and a search for the cause is initiated.

A sensory neuropathy may be caused by diabetes mellitus, chronic alcoholism, pernicious anemia, drug intoxication, chronic renal failure (uremia) and hypothyroidism. This list is not complete. Identification of the disease producing the neuropathy makes the treatment of that disease possible and improvement in the symptoms will result. Residual numbness may persist, however, but general improvement can be expected.

MOTOR

The facial weakness of Bell's palsy is mentioned in chapter 2. Although they suggest a stroke, the signs of Bell's palsy are not representative of a stroke. Peroneal and radial nerve palsies (see below) also may be mistaken for a stroke. Motor neuropathies, other than peroneal and radial nerve palsies, may occur, predominantly affecting the feet and legs. Only after several months might the hands and arms become involved. These neuropathies are characterized by weakness and, as time progresses, wasting away of the muscles may be evident. These symptoms might suggest amyotrophic lateral sclerosis and other degenerative muscle diseases (see chapter 15). Sensorimotor neuropathy, to be discussed later, includes those diseases that are responsible for motor neuropathies.

Peroneal Nerve Palsy

Many of us sit with our legs crossed. After a period of time we usually shift and cross our legs the opposite way. In cramped quarters such as a car or plane, reshifting may not be possible. Under such conditions, perhaps after a three-hour trip, you get up, start to walk and one leg feels "funny." One foot drags the ground with each step. The following day, things are no better; the foot continues to drag and you can't pick it up. The rest of your leg is strong; only your ankle is weak. Could this be a stroke? No. You have compressed a peroneal nerve by prolonged crossing of your legs. Certainly these symptoms would suggest the possibility of a stroke, and you may want to see your physician to be sure you haven't had one. Simply knowing that you haven't had a stroke is worthwhile.

Recovery from peroneal nerve palsy usually occurs in eight to ten weeks. No medication is necessary and there is no residual effect. Remember that if this has occurred once, it suggests that the peroneal nerve is easily compressed by crossing your legs.

Radial Nerve Palsy

The radial nerve, among other functions, bends our wrist and extends our fingers. It circles around the bone in the upper arm on its course down into the forearm. You may have fallen asleep on the couch or in a chair and, unknown to you, your upper arm leaned heavily against the edge of your resting place. Upon awakening you notice that you can't extend your wrist and you can't even pick up a glass. You have compressed the radial nerve during your sleep. The arm seems weak, but in reality everything works well except your wrist. This again could be interpreted as a stroke. See your physician. Recovery from this condition as well as from peroneal nerve palsy occurs in most cases within eight to ten weeks without medication or other treatment. The use of a splint to support the wrist is helpful.

MIXED NEUROPATHY
(Motor and Sensory)

Not all neuropathies are clearly motor or sensory; both components may be present, therefore the term "sensorimotor neuropathies." The Guillain-Barré syndrome is predominantly a motor neuropathy even though there may be some sensory symptoms present. The Guillain-Barré syndrome occurs in all age groups. A few years ago, several cases occurred that were presumably caused by flu vaccinations. The disease often is preceded by nausea, vomiting and diarrhea or sore throat and cough. However, there may not be any antecedent symptoms. Usually the flu is the flu and nothing else occurs; however, if Guillain-Barré syndrome is to develop, it does so within one or two weeks after the appearance of flulike symptoms. A feeling of unexplained weakness occurs. Your exercise tolerance is decreased. Walking a block may be impossible. A distorted sensation of numbness, tingling or crawling may occur in your legs. Your arms are now weak and even holding them over your head is a real feat. This generalized weakness comes over you over a period of seven days. Just think of yourself regressing from a state of normal strength to barely being able to get around in such a short period of time! This disease moves fast and you should too—to your physician. This disease becomes life threatening when the respiratory muscles become involved, usually within the first fourteen days. Attention to your breathing is vital. Most patients survive this

45

disease with support provided for their respiratory system. Almost all hospitals have the capability of providing respiratory support. There should be no failure on your part in recognizing this sudden loss of muscle strength. This disease is self-limited and, with adequate respiratory care, functional recovery can be expected. In fact, most patients can expect full recovery, but a very small percentage may develop a chronic relapsing form of the disease.

There are many other causes of peripheral neuropathies. Diabetes mellitus is one of the more common and usually manifests itself later in life. Chronic alcoholism, pernicious anemia and uremia are also relatively frequent causes. I mention this because someone, somewhere will be helped in identifying the cause for his or her pheripheral neuropathy if the list is inclusive enough. Poisoning with heavy metals such as lead or arsenic may cause a peripheral neuropathy. Neuropathies may be associated with cancer and on occasion precede the onset of the malignancy. Hypothyroidism may be associated with a peripheral neuropathy. Some neuropathies are inherited, and knowledge of your family history of disease is most important. Some drugs such as Furadantin and Vincristine have been implicated in the development of peripheral neuropathy.

Peripheral neuropathies are danger signals that indicate a generalized disease may be present or some medication may be causing the symptoms. Neuropathies are *not* part of aging. Get an answer to the problem.

Peripheral Neuropathy

CHECKLIST

THE symptoms of peripheral neuropathies are signals to you that an undiagnosed disease is present or that medications you are taking have caused the symptoms.

1. Have you recently noticed numbness of your toes and feet?

2. Have you noticed that the numbness (toes and feet) is now above your ankles?

3. Do your fingertips feel like sandpaper?

4. Do you have difficulty feeling and manipulating objects with your hands?

5. Does one foot seem to slap the ground when you walk?

6. Do you have difficulty in putting on your shoe because you can't flex your foot?

7. Do you have difficulty picking up a glass when the rest of your arm seems strong?

8. Have you developed a rapid, general weakness?

8. Tardive Dyskinesia

TARDIVE dyskinesias are abnormal involuntary movements induced by certain medications. The appearance of these movements usually occurs only after several weeks of treatment, hence the term "tardive," or tending toward delayed development. Why should tardive dyskinesias be discussed? Because the aging population is at greater risk for the development of these movement disorders.

The medications implicated in this problem are, in general, major tranquilizers. Medications of this nature were developed initially to treat patients with serious psychiatric disorders, and in many instances the patients became more manageable. As time passed, the usage of these medications was extended to treat problems other than those of a primarily psychiatric nature; problems such as, "Doc, is there anything you can give him to make him sleep? He's up all hours of the night." Or, "She's always had a quick temper, but during the past six months she's been blowing up more frequently." Situations of the nature described and many, many more are annoying to the people involved and often require treatment. Tranquilizers would appear to serve this purpose; they have been used and are being used.

Not all patients over the age of sixty who take

tranquilizers will develop tardive dyskinesias. Not all patients over the age of sixty who take tranquilizers will develop drug-induced Parkinsonism (see page 87). However, there is a risk, and it increases with age.

There are several movement disorders associated with tardive dyskinesias and I will explain each separately.

Buccal-Lingual (Cheek-Tongue)

The buccal-lingual movements that may occur are facial grimacing, protrusion of the tongue, pouting, sucking and involuntary grunts. These movements are uncontrollable, unsightly and unpleasant to others. As a result, the sufferer avoids social situations and tends to become reclusive.

Blepharospasm

Blepharospasm, forcible eye closure, may accompany facial grimacing or it may occur independently. This action is also uncontrollable and may last (eyes closed) for several seconds. If this should occur as you are driving, it could be disastrous.

Akathisia

Akathisia, a restlessness different from the restless legs syndrome, may occur (see page 14). This compulsion to move about occurs during the waking day and one is literally forced to get up and walk or pace about. On occasion an uncontrollable rocking motion may occur while sitting. There may be involuntary movements of the arms and legs, which resemble but differ from the tremor of Parkinson's disease. These movements are quick and make one appear to have total body fidgets; sometimes these movements may be confused with a condition called Huntington's chorea. All of the movements described may occur independently or in conjunction with each other.

Knowing that such side effects can occur with the use of certain tranquilizers, particularly in those over sixty, should make you wary of taking them. If you are taking any of the medications listed below, and have noticed any unusual movements, stop the medication and consult your physician.

The movements of tardive dyskinesia may disappear within three to four weeks after discontinuing the medication. This does not always happen; the movements still may persist. There is no treatment, to my knowledge, that will effectively treat all persistent tardive dyskinesias.

Here are some of the more commonly used tranquilizers that can produce tardive dyskinesias in susceptible people:

Compazine
Haldol
Loxitane
Navane

Prolixin
Thorazine
Triavil

When sedatives or tranquilizers are prescribed for you, *always* ask about side effects. If another medication can be prescribed that does not carry the risk of tardive dyskinesia, request it. Use the term "tardive dyskinesia" specifically when asking about side effects.

CHECKLIST

You have been given a new prescription to settle your nerves. The doctor is in a hurry and you forget to ask about any side effects. Over the next few weeks one of the following problems might develop; if so, tell your physician.

1. Tremor of a hand or foot

2. Stiffness or lack of mobility

3. Loss of facial expression

4. Restless—can't sit still—must get up and move

5. Involuntary facial movements, noticed by friends

6. Your eyes close and you have difficulty opening them

9. Myasthenia Gravis

MYASTHENIA gravis is a neuromuscular disease caused by a block in the transmissions of the nerve impulse to a muscle, which results in weakness. Muscles may be affected in the arms, legs, chest, face, eyes and pharynx (the swallowing mechanism). The disease occurs most commonly in the under-sixty age group; however, its onset after the age of sixty is not unusual.

Myasthenia gravis is a "sneaky" disease in that symptoms frequently go unnoticed for several weeks. How can this be? The neuromuscular block becomes most apparent after exercise. Minimal activity produces modest weakness, whereas normal activity will make the symptoms more apparent. The activities that I am speaking of are walking, talking, chewing and keeping your eyes open. In patients over the age of sixty the disease frequently restricts itself to the eye muscles and chewing-swallowing muscles.

A droopy eyelid (ptosis) frequently heralds the onset of myasthenia gravis, and usually is more apparent as the day progresses. This symptom comes and goes, as do so many neurological symptoms, and is more evident some days than others. The droopy eyelid may occur on one or both sides. As some people age, their eyes become puffy and they appear to squint. The droopy lid may impair vision and the eyelid needs to be raised with a finger to permit vision. Double vision may occur in conjunction with the droopy lid and will also become more evident as the day progresses. Now comes the dilemma. You've noticed the double vision and droopy eyelid; you're in the age group for a stroke and you consult your physician. Your time perception for the duration of the symptoms may be hazy. Has it been a month or just a few days? You do have high blood pressure, although it seems to be well controlled. The initial impression may well be "a little stroke." During the next two weeks you begin to have difficulty swallowing, and your jaws tire when you chew your food at dinnertime. Could this be considered an extension of your stroke? You bet it could. Now, you have a CAT head scan, the result of which is normal. Remember, strokes usually do their job in twenty-four to thirty-six hours. Occasionally the time frame is longer, but not very often.

Remember, the importance of onset and duration of symptoms is *vital* in establishing diagnoses in diseases of the nervous system. Physicians aren't magicians; they need your help in symptom identification, and only *you* have been a witness to the progression of your symptoms. There isn't a thing wrong with saying, "Doc, do you think I might have myasthenia gravis?" It is refreshing to me when patients suggest a diagnostic possibility that could well be right. It indicates that they are interested in themselves and knowledgeable about their condition. Moreover, if they can help to establish a diagnosis of their condition, we can stop searching and start treating.

The symptoms of double vision, droopy eyelid and difficulty in swallowing and chewing are the most frequently found symptoms of myasthenia gravis in the over-sixty population. In younger people, generalized weakness and breathing problems in addition to the above symptoms are also present. These problems almost always follow the symptoms first mentioned.

On occasion a tumor in the chest, usually benign, called a thymoma, may be responsible for myasthenia gravis. This is operable, and removal of the tumor will improve the myasthenic condition.

Another condition that starts with a single droopy eyelid and double vision needs to be mentioned. The symptoms develop over a short period of time, four or five days. They do not fluctuate and are associated with pain in the eye. These symptoms are caused by an aneurysm and indicate a serious problem. It is imperative that you see your physician. Many aneurysms are operable and correctable with current neurosurgical techniques.

Certain tests are available that assist in making the diagnosis of myasthenia gravis. The simplest test is the Tensilon test, which involves an intravenous injection of Tensilon. For example, if a patient has a droopy eyelid and the eye opens within seconds after the injection, he has tested positively for myasthenia gravis. Other tests include an antibody study of the blood that is 85 percent accurate (leaving 15 percent of patients undiagnosed) and an electromyogram (EMG) study of muscles. These tests may be positive *only* when symptoms are present, so make your appointment to see your physician for the time of the day when your symptoms are usually present. This will most often be in the afternoon, when the droopy lid and/or double vision can be identified. Medications are available for the management of myasthenia gravis once the diagnosis is established. Think about myasthenia gravis if your eyelid becomes droopy and you have double vision.

CHECKLIST

REMEMBER, the symptoms of myasthenia gravis become more apparent as the day progresses.

1. Have you had difficulty chewing and swallowing your evening meal?

2. Have you been able to eat the next day's breakfast without difficulty?

3. Has someone noticed in the late afternoon that one of your eyelids was droopy?

4. Have you noticed double vision in the afternoon that regularly clears by the next morning?

10. Alcoholism

IT is not surprising that there are older people suffering from alcoholism. The seduction probably began years earlier with the cocktail hour and has now evolved into a way of life. Many people enjoy two or three drinks before dinner and even have wine with dinner. In general, they manage their drinking habits, although they may well be at risk for subsequent alcoholism.

Sixty-five-year-old alcoholics have had years of experience. There are few short-term alcoholics—longevity seems to play an important role. Young alcoholics, teenagers who persist in drinking, will not reach the age of sixty-five because they'll die from the complications of alcoholism: trauma (physical abuse, gunshot or vehicular), exposure to the elements (pneumonia, freezing) or the organic complications of alcoholism—cirrhosis of the liver and degenerative changes in the nervous system. So alcoholics in the aging population were not alcoholics at the age of fifteen or sixteen. They are the people of the traditional cocktail hour who, after years of practice, elect to forgo dinner and have a few extra drinks, or those whose three-martini lunch carries into the cocktail hour and into oblivion.

Women in the over-sixty age group are at great risk for developing alcoholism. They may be widows or they may have husbands who continue to work and/or have continuing hobbies and interests. The children are gone and their nurturing years are over. They may feel less and less useful, and they most likely feel the loss of attractiveness that comes with age. They have time on their hands, which easily breeds discontent and misery. Misery loves company and in this particular situation, company isn't hard to find—it's so easy to talk over a drink. The occasional social drinker can, under these circumstances, be easily led down the path to chronic alcoholism.

It is surprising the tolerance that some people seem to have for alcohol. For years they may function well in responsible jobs, but ultimately the liver and/or nervous system begins to show the effects. Why one develops cirrhosis of the liver rather than degenerative changes of the nervous system or vice versa is not known. A genetic predisposition for developing one and/or the other probably plays a role.

The socioeconomic implications of chronic alcoholism are well known. Divorce, loss of work and alienation of family and friends are the most usual consequences. Anyone who drinks is aware of the problems of alcoholism, but such knowledge doesn't deter the thousands who join the ranks of alcoholics every year. Most alcoholics are aware that liver disease may result from their drinking; few are aware of the serious neurological complications that may occur. Some people cause their own destruction with little apparent concern. Yet if they knew that they might develop an intolerable burning in their feet, a weakness that makes it difficult to walk, hallucinatory experiences, blackouts, withdrawal seizures, unsteadiness that prevents walking, double vision, memory lapses and impotence, they might take a second look at their drinking habits.

Impotence in the alcoholic male, whether under or over sixty, is a relatively common occurrence. Over the age of sixty, sexual drive tends to lessen and under these circumstances, a little alcohol goes a long way. Alcohol in this situation dictates that there will be no activity. This doesn't make for a happy home, but it can be corrected—by abstinence from alcohol.

Chronic alcoholism has been mentioned as a cause of peripheral neuropathy. The symptoms usually develop over several months: numbness, tingling, burning, weakness and loss of muscle mass. These symptoms initially begin in the feet and legs; ultimately the hands and arms may become involved. Walking may be impossible because of pain and weakness. Recovery of function is possible with cessation of drinking, improved diet, taking vitamins and time—several weeks to months. If these symptoms are left unattended for several months, recovery is improbable.

"Terrific party. Who drove home?"

"You did."

"I did?"

Blackouts are not uncommon among alcoholics. They may function in a reasonably normal fashion during the blackout, but will have no recollection of events that transpired over a particular period of time. Certainly the first experience with a blackout should temper one's drinking, but unfortunately this is not always the case.

Seizures may occur when one is actively drinking, but they more often occur when an attempt is made to stop drinking, hence the name "withdrawal seizures." Several seizures may occur during the immediate withdrawal period that could be life threatening. An illness requiring hospitalization may induce withdrawal from alcohol by virtue of the confinement. The potential for a serious problem is present both for the patient and for the physician. For instance, a heavy drinker, not recognized as an alcoholic, who has had in the past six months several blackout spells, has an attack of appendicitis. He is operated on, and does well for two days following surgery. The third day, however, he has several seizures for no apparent reason. He then becomes confused, belligerent, hallucinatory and combative. The patient is confused and the physician is confused by this unexpected course. Now the patient's wife tells the doctor that her husband has been a heavy drinker. The explanation is clear: the patient has had withdrawal seizures and delerium tremens. Death can result from delerium tremens. What should have been an uncomplicated appendectomy has turned into a horror story.

Intellectual deterioration, poor judgment, faulty memory, sloppy habits—these symptoms will sound familiar when you read about dementia in chapter 15. The heavy drinker (alcoholic) may arrive at this sorry state of affairs. Once successful, he or she is now in essence nonfunctional.

You may have noticed that your next-door neighbor, the one with the perpetual parties, is using a cane when walking. He seems to think all right, but his speech is slurred and his walking is bad. He is developing a selective degeneration of the brain, which maintains our posture and coordinates muscle action involved in our movements. His gait disorder, ataxia, may progress to the point where he will be unable to walk.

Some alcoholics develop, in addition to the gait disorder, double vision, confusion and memory impairment. These symptoms are called the Wernicke-Korsakoff Syndrome, a formidable name for a formidable disease.

Tremor that could be confused with the tremor of Parkinson's disease occurs in alcoholism. The tremor involves the hands and many times spreads up the arms so that there appears to be a generalized shaking of the body. The tremor is most apparent during early withdrawal from alcohol. The tremor responds to a few stiff drinks, and the show is on the road again. Withdrawal from alcohol has to be a terrible experience, but not as bad as the permanent neurological problems associated with continued drinking.

Anyone who drinks should be aware of the consequences of alcoholism, especially its serious side effects on the nervous system. If you drink and have any of the problems discussed in this chapter, what should you do? See your physician and get confirmation of the problem. There is no sure way to stop drinking but many avenues are available: Alcoholics Anonymous, Al-anon, alcohol rehabilitation units, counselors, clergy and friends. Whatever it takes, get involved and cure the problem.

CHECKLIST

MILLIONS of people fit into the category of social drinkers, yet sometimes they drink too much. The following questions will help you decide whether you have an alcohol problem.

1. Do you have persistent numbness and tingling in your feet?

2. Have you developed an intolerable burning in your feet?

3. Have you ever had a seizure while giving up or after you gave up alcohol?

4. Have you forgotten an important social or business engagement?

5. Does your balance seem to be "off," and does it affect your walking?

6. Have you recently had a blackout associated with a night out?

11. Seizures

A seizure may occur in any age group, and it is usually evident as a convulsion. If you're at a shopping center, and suddenly you fall to the floor, lose consciousness and have jerking of the arms and legs, it certainly attracts attention. An ambulance is called, and a quick trip to the emergency room is made. Witnesses verify the incident and a seizure disorder is suspected.

Under these circumstances, you would be hospitalized and a battery of tests would be ordered in an attempt to identify the cause of the seizure. Seizures are symptomatic of underlying brain irritability and may express themselves in many ways other than by a convulsion. All seizures are not associated with loss of consciousness. However, your awareness of your surroundings may be impaired.

Seizures are diagnosed by the description of events that have occurred. The electroencephalogram (EEG) may be beneficial in confirming the diagnosis, but, in many patients the EEG may be normal even in the presence of a documented seizure disorder. Here again your symptoms are more reliable in establishing a diagnosis.

Sensory Seizures

A few years ago I saw a man who complained of numbness in one of his legs. His symptoms had begun twelve years before he came to me. Initially, he had noticed numbness in his big toe. The numbness lasted for about thirty seconds and occurred once or twice a month. The months went by and then two, three years passed. By then the foot and then the ankle became involved. The duration of the numbness remained about the same, however. The frequency of attacks increased to four or five times a month. At the time I saw him, the entire leg was affected and the attacks were occurring daily. These attacks were sensory seizures and were ignored by the patient for years. This man had a brain tumor that was causing the seizures. Fortunately, it was benign. Sensory seizures are brief in duration, lasting between thirty seconds and two minutes. They occur spontaneously, and when they end, people function in their normal fashion. Sensory seizures are subjective; they are only felt by you, and obviously, they can't be seen. These seizures can involve any part of the body, and the sensation can be interpreted as numbness, tingling, itching, burning or crawling.

Focal Motor Seizures

These seizures may involve the face, arm or leg. They are termed "focal" because only part of the body is involved. A convulsion may start as a focal motor seizure; eventually it becomes generalized, involving both arms and legs, and then consciousness is lost. The focal motor seizures we are concerned with do not involve the loss of consciousness. The seizure can vary from a light twitching of the hand to a jerking motion of the entire extremity. The jerking or twitching is usually rhythmic; it begins suddenly and ends suddenly. The duration, as with sensory seizures, is brief, lasting for seconds, or a minute or two at most.

The first reaction to a focal motor seizure will probably be, "What was that?" It shouldn't be attributed to fatigue, having a bad day, or "maybe these things happen when you get older." The seizures tend to recur in a stereotyped manner, although the frequency varies. A convulsion will get you prompt medical attention. Focal motor seizures will attract only your attention and again the burden lies with you in recognizing that something is wrong. Certainly after three or four events you should seek medical advice.

Complex Partial Seizures

Complex partial seizures were originally described as psychomotor or temporal lobe seizures. So that you may more easily understand what happens during one of these seizures, I'll call them an "experience." The experience is totally subjective; that is, the event that occurs during the seizure is *only* experienced by the patient, and, to the patient, the event is always identical. Some seizure-related events that have been experienced in the patient's unawareness are hearing a familiar song, hearing a tape recorder whirling backward, seeing a familiar room, seeing an unfamiliar room, smelling a foul odor and feeling a sense of impending doom or profound depression. These events recur in the same manner with each experience. During the time the seizure is occurring the person is unable to communicate and does not understand conversations. Associated with the experience may be some motor activities such as lip smacking, purposeless movements of the hand such as picking at one's clothing, shuffling papers or patting an object. These "spells" may occur for months before some people become fully aware that something is wrong. Don't be one of these people. Don't be unaware.

Nocturnal Seizures

Many seizures occur only at night or in the early morning hours. I am now referring to a major motor seizure or convulsion. Your bed partner will awaken and undoubtedly observe part of the seizure. If you sleep alone, the only awareness of something having happened may be a sore tongue (from being bitten) or perhaps a wet bed due to urinary incontinence. One patient with nocturnal seizures saw her physician after she had awakened on two occasions with a bleeding tongue. She was told that her tongue was too big!

Myoclonic Jerks

We have all experienced a sudden jerking of the body at just about the time we're falling asleep, a "startle" reaction, as it were. This is a natural occurrence. This sudden jerking, usually involving an arm, may occur during the daytime, and if it does, it's termed a "myoclonic jerk." A most vivid example occurs when you're brushing your teeth. If the jerk occurs, the arm goes up and the toothbrush is thrown! These myoclonic jerks may occur as an isolated phenomenon or they may herald the onset of a convulsion. The first two or three experiences may be ignored or dismissed as odd occurrences. They *are not* normal and should be investigated.

Post-Stroke Seizures

It's bad enough to have a stroke; it's worse luck yet to have seizures after a stroke. A small number of post-stroke patients have seizures; I mention this because many patients do not realize that seizures can be managed effectively with medication. I recently saw a seventy-three-year-old man who had had a stroke three months prior to my seeing him. The stroke left him with some residual weakness of his left arm, but his left leg had good functional recovery. The problem: he was having difficulty walking, and at the time I saw him he was using a walker. He told me that his left leg just "gave out." How did this happen? The leg would jerk three or four times and wouldn't support him. This had been happening five or six times daily. He was treated with Dilantin, the seizures stopped, and he no longer needs the walker. Any of the types of seizures here may occur as post-stroke seizures.

It has been estimated that seizures occur in non-hospitalized elderly patients at the rate of four per thousand. If there are 25 to 30 million people over sixty-five, that would mean one hundred thousand patients annually. What causes seizures in those over sixty? According to information published in the *Journal of the American Medical Association,* 30 percent were related to strokes, 8 percent to head trauma, 2 percent to brain tumors, 10 percent to drug or alcohol withdrawal and 50 percent to unknown causes. Many medications are available for the control of seizures, and these are well known to virtually all physicians.

Perhaps you have experienced one of the several types seizures described. This is not your imagination, or is it? After the fourth occurrence you see your doctor. An EEG (electroencephalogram) is performed and the result is normal. Many doctors will dismiss the possibility of a seizure disorder on the basis of a normal EEG. Your doctor suggests the possibility of a transient ischemic attack or a little stroke—not a bad suggestion—and orders the appropriate laboratory tests. The CAT scan is normal; no evidence of a stroke or tumor is found. No diagnosis, no treatment. What then?

You are still suspicious that you may have a seizure disorder. Now is the time to request a consultation with a neurologist. If your doctor is reluctant to do this, call the local medical society and ask for the name and address of a neurologist near your community. You might also call for an appointment in the neurology outpatient services of your local medical school.

When you see the neurologist, he will need to review your EEG and CAT scan. He finds them to be normal. You then relate your history of events to him and the diagnosis of a seizure disorder, in all probability, will be confirmed by your history.

Do seizures mean that you have a bad brain? No. Why do seizures occur? Most seizures result from unusual electrical activity in a small number of brain cells. Different symptoms occur, depending upon the location of these cells in the brain. Because of the specific location of these cells, the motor, sensory, visual, etc., symptoms that are produced are virtually identical with each experience.

Medications used in the treatment of seizures suppress the unusual brain activity and control the seizure symptoms. The cause of the seizure is not cured by the medication.

Seizures can be a difficult diagnostic problem that frequently requires the services of a neurologist. Once the diagnosis is established and the medication is prescribed, your family physician can effectively manage the problem. Most patients can expect a decrease in the frequency of their seizures with appropriate medication and some will also be seizure-free.

One fact that is mentioned throughout this book and cannot be repeated too often is that *you* must recognize events that are changes from your usual state of health. Often different events are attributed to "getting older." We can't change getting older, but we can change the course of our illnesses.

CHECKLIST

SEIZURES are brief in duration, may occur at any time and, with the exception of a convulsion, you function in your normal manner after the spell.

The following questions will refresh your memory for these events.

1. Has your face, or an arm, or a leg suddenly become numb, then within a minute or two felt perfectly normal?

2. Has your face, a foot, leg, hand or arm suddenly started twitching or jerking and just as suddenly stopped?

3. Has someone asked you, "What's the matter?" and you then remember an unusual feeling or experience that has just happened?

4. Has your arm suddenly jerked, causing you to drop or throw what you had in your hand?

5. Has your spouse awakened you to tell you that you were moaning and jerking in your sleep?

12. Stroke

STROKE is a major medical problem for those over fifty-five. There are approximately five hundred thousand occurrences of stroke annually in the United States. The greatest number of strokes occur in the over-sixty age group. Predisposing factors for the risk of stroke include high blood pressure, diabetes mellitus and elevated cholesterol and blood lipid levels. Control of these problems with medication and diet decreases the risk of stroke. Yet many people are lax about regulating their diet and regularly taking their medication. This casual attitude and loss of control can lead to disaster. We can be our own worst enemy or best friend.

Many, many people have strokes who are not in the high-risk groups and who appear to be enjoying good health. Even so, frequently there are signs and symptoms that may herald a forthcoming stroke. Identifying these signs and symptoms is important. The old adage "An ounce of prevention is worth a pound of cure" still holds true. Strokes may be caused by a brain hemorrhage, a thrombus (clot) or by showers of tiny fragments (emboli) that block small vessels.

The most usual site for the development of a thrombotic stroke lies in the common carotid artery, which can be felt pulsating in your neck. Materials build up on the wall of the artery to form a clot. This clot obstructs the flow of blood, or tiny fragments from the clot may block other blood vessels. If the blood supply to an area of the brain is partially blocked and then cleared, symptoms may last only minutes or up to several hours. These events are called transient ischemic (diminished blood supply) attacks. These attacks produce symptoms that give us clues to the possibility of a stroke in the future. Transient ischemic attacks tend to be recurring and each recurrence is almost identical to the preceding one. Now let us look at the signs and symptoms produced by transient ischemic attacks.

Visual Disturbances

Amaurosis fugax literally means transient blindness. This occurs suddenly, with no warning. The vision in one eye dims as if a veil has been dropped. Within a few seconds the vision is obscured. In a matter of minutes the veil rises and vision returns. Loss of vision, even for a few minutes, should be impressive. I have seen people who have had several attacks of amaurosis fugax before they sought medical advice. This symptom is a classic one for transient ischemic attacks and is recognized by most physicians as such. If it occurs, check it out.

"Visual field cut" (hemianopia) happens suddenly and with no warning. Suddenly you realize that you see nothing to your left (or right, as the case may be). This visual field cut may last for minutes or up to several hours. Strangely, I have seen patients with this problem who were unaware of its existence until they walked straight into a door or bumped into someone. Transient visual field cut, not symptomatic of a stroke, can occur in conjunction with migraine headaches, usually preceding the headache. As one gets older, the visual field cut in migraine may continue to recur; however, the headache may no longer occur.

"Double vision" (diplopia) is another symptom that may be transient and recurring. This may happen with near vision while reading, with far vision such as looking down the highway, and when you look to the right or left. Double vision may make objects appear side by side or one on top of another.

Numbness (Paresthesias)

Almost everybody has had numbness or tingling in some part of the body at some time in his life. For instance, upon awaking in the morning, your arm is numb. You rub and shake it and in a few minutes the sensation is gone. After sitting with your legs crossed, one leg is numb and, in like manner, the numbness is gone within a few minutes. We are not concerned with these kinds of numbness.

Almost everyone has a different appreciation of the sensation of numbness. It has been variously described to me as the feeling after the dentist has injected an anesthetic, tingling, itching, crawling, burning, heavy, wooden and dead.

Transient numbness, sudden in onset and without provocation, may occur only in an arm or leg or both. It may occur just on one side of your face or may involve your face and hand. On occasion it may "split the body in half." Numbness around the lips only may also occur. These symptoms may occur independently or in combinations. Repeated attacks that clear up, leaving no symptoms, suggest transient ischemic attacks.

Weakness (Paresis)

A change in your muscle strength may vary from paralysis to the loss of fine motor control in a hand or foot. If the weakness is profound, it can hardly escape notice. The other gradations of weakness need your attention. Tripping over a carpet, stumbling when ascending stairs or stepping up on a curbing should not be attributed to being awkward or getting older. A feeling of heaviness in an arm that results in spilling a cup of coffee, dropping an object or being unable to open a jar shouldn't be accepted as just having a bad day.

A loss of strength in your facial muscles is quite obvious. For instance, you look into the mirror and one side of your face sags. You smile and on one side your lips don't respond. What was once a fairly symmetrical face is no more. This change may be due to a transient ischemic attack—or to a condition known as Bell's palsy, which is described in chapter 2. These changes in your normal strength, lasting minutes to hours with subsequent returns to normal function, must *not* be ignored.

Amnesia

You remember watching the noon news and now it is almost three o'clock. What happened between twelve o'clock and three? You may have experienced "global" amnesia and registered no incoming events for that period of time. During that time you may have functioned in an apparently normal fashion, and you only become aware of the time lapse when you are unable to recall events that must have or should have occurred in that time. This experience has to be disturbing, and you should let someone know about it. This symptom is difficult to explain and even your physician may suggest that you simply dozed off. If it occurs a second time, which it probably will, *don't give up* until you get a diagnosis.

Speech Disturbances

Your speech may become slurred or sloppy and your tongue just doesn't seem to work right (dysarthria). Words become scrambled, and you can't remember or find the right word to say. Your conversation doesn't make sense to the people around you (aphasia). Suddenly, after a period of time, you are able to communicate in your usual fashion. This again is a memorable experience. It should get your attention and direct you to your physician.

The transient experiences of weakness, numbness, amnesia, visual symptoms and speech problems are telling you something: you may be having transient ischemic attacks. These attacks are almost always sudden in onset. This *sudden* change from your previous health should alert you to a problem. Too often these symptoms are ignored or attributed to getting older. If the symptom occurs only once and is brief in duration, this attitude is understandable. Often there will be repeat performances and a longer duration of symptoms. Once they have your attention, what should you do?

How you describe your symptoms to your physician is of utmost importance in making the diagnosis. What happened? When did it happen? Was this the first experience? How long did it last? How did it go away? How did you feel after it was gone? You may have a head scan (CAT) or you may have laboratory work performed, and the results will be normal. What then? You may have an arteriogram, a study of the blood vessels, done. A radiologist injects dye into the blood vessels that go through the neck to the brain. These studies may show a blockage in an artery that is decreasing blood flow to the brain; or they may show a smaller clot that has ulcerated. From these findings your physician will determine whether an operation is indicated. If no blockage is shown, blood thinners, aspirin or other medications may be used to facilitate circulation.

You helped in identifying the problem and, by having treatment instituted, prevented a stroke from occurring. If diagnostic techniques for studying blood vessels are not available in your community, you should request referral to a place that can perform them. If you feel that your request for a referral will hurt your doctor's feelings, remember that hurting someone's feelings is far less important that hurting your own body. You can also call your county or state medical society for referrals.

If you are unfortunate and have a stroke, what then? Recovery from a stroke varies from virtually complete recovery to paralysis and inability to communicate. Most stroke patients fall somewhere in between, with partial return of function. A major problem that is frequently overlooked in the care of a stroke patient is depression. Who wouldn't be depressed, having to deal with the loss or partial loss of function of an arm or leg? Each of us handles problems like this in our own style, and our styles vary from, "I'm going to lick this," to "I'm going to lie down and die." The choice lies with the individual.

Many people deny their depression and resist attempts by friends and associates to help them. Through hell and high water they are going to stay down. Although antidepressant medications do not "cure," they can be beneficial in helping you over the rough spots and should be used. Don't be timid about requesting these medications from your physician.

Remember, any of the symptoms mentioned in this chapter that are sudden in onset, brief in duration, clear spontaneously, tend to repeat themselves and depart from your general health should *not* be ignored. See your physician. Your role in diagnosing the possibility of transient ischemic attacks is vital, and may, with medications or surgery, forestall or prevent a future stroke.

CHECKLIST

WHEN you compare this chapter and checklist with the chapter on seizures, you will notice many similarities. The identification of a transient ischemic attack versus a seizure is dependent on the information you tell your doctor.

Transient ischemic attacks may last for several minutes or for hours. Seizures usually last from thirty seconds to one or two minutes.

The first episode will take you by surprise. The second episode gives you the opportunity to time it.

Seizures usually are of short duration. The symptoms of transient ischemic attacks may disappear in minutes or hours, but ever so slight numbness, tingling and weakness may last hours longer.

A convulsion will often be followed by confusion for several minutes or up to a half hour. Seizures without loss of consciousness produce confusion during the seizure. You are your normal self within minutes.

1. Have you experienced visual loss as if a shade were drawn? Have you experienced double vision near or far away? Have you walked into a door, sofa or other objects because you didn't see them?

2. Have you had one or more attacks of numbness (dead, wooden, tingling, heavy) involving an arm or leg, or one side of the body or face?

3. Have you tripped or stumbled, then later realized that your leg was weak?

4. Have you had difficulty pushing open a door that usually opens easily? Does it seem heavy? Is one of your arms weak?

5. You remember turning on the television set to watch the football game. Suddenly it is half-time. What happened?

6. Has your speech become slurred during a conversation, then not understandable at all to your companion?

If any of these situations have occurred, write them down in detail, then see your doctor.

13. Parkinson's Disease

PARKINSON'S disease occurs predominantly in people over the age of sixty. The percentage of cases under the age of sixty would be less than 5 percent. There are approximately a half million cases of Parkinson's disease in the United States and approximately fifty thousand new cases are diagnosed each year, according to Cecil's *Textbook of Medicine.*

Most of us would recognize a person with advanced Parkinson's disease: the stooped posture, shuffling gait, tremulous hands and the soft monotonous voice. Dr. Parkinson termed it the "shaking palsy" in 1871. But before reaching this stage, many subtle changes occur: the information here will enable you to identify them and increase the likelihood of early diagnosis.

Early diagnosis of all treatable diseases enables therapy to be initiated to control symptoms. Obviously, controlling your symptoms makes you more functional. If a diagnosis is made late in the course of a disease, when irremediable changes have already occurred, the disease may not respond as well to treatment.

I recently saw a sixty-eight-year-old woman in the hospital to evaluate a hand tremor. She had been admitted and operated on for a fractured hip; the fractured hip was the result of a fall. She told me that she had fallen ten or twelve times during the preceding year. What caused her to fall so often? She didn't know, but responded, "I'm just getting older, you know." I'm amazed at how friends and family will accept this explanation of symptoms and pay no further attention. This woman had Parkinson's disease and her symptoms dated back at least one year. If only a diagnosis could have been made and treatment instituted, a fractured hip might well have been prevented.

The classic symptoms of Parkinson's disease are tremor, rigidity and bradykinesia. Briefly, tremor may be described as a shaking, quivering or a restless feeling. Rigidity is most often described as a stiffness. The most colorful description I've been given for rigidity was, "Doc, I think I need a shot of grease." Bradykinesia literally means slow movement. These three symptoms, all being present, constitute the picture of full-blown Parkinson's disease. Each will be discussed more fully in this chapter.

The one feature of Parkinson's disease most often recognized by physicians is the tremor, but the tremor isn't always present early in the course of the disease. Most important, only one of the triad of symptoms may be present initially. Also of great importance, the symptom may appear only on one side.

Tremor

Tremor of the hand caused by Parkinson's disease occurs at rest, when you're relaxed. You may first notice the tremor in your thumb and index finger. This symptom, as with all other symptoms of Parkinson's disease, may be more evident some days than others before it becomes permanent. Tremor of the hand, best noted by a companion, is also frequently present when you're walking. However, it tends to diminish when you stand still. Tremor of the foot may occur independently or in conjunction with tremor of the hand. This is noticeable only when sitting and frequently escapes observation.

Tremors *Not* Related to Parkinson's Disease

There is another tremor that occurs independently of Parkinson's disease. This tremor frequently occurs before the age of sixty and may well have been present for years. The tremor is evident when initiating action, not while at rest, as in Parkinson's disease. Drinking a glass of wine or a highball may cause the tremor to disappear. This tremor is called "essential" or "familial" and differs in its treatment from Parkinson's disease. Occasionally associated with this tremor is a to-and-fro or nodding movement of the head and neck. Frequently there is a family history of similar tremor, and this should be brought to the physician's attention. The duration of the tremor in the absence of rigidity and bradykinesia should tell you and your physician that this is *not* Parkinson's disease.

Other tremors that may be misdiagnosed as Parkinson's disease deserve your attention. Diagnosis dictates treatment; if the wrong diagnosis is made, the treatment will obviously fail.

Chronic alcoholism may produce a tremor and unsteadiness when walking. These symptoms could easily be misinterpreted as Parkinson's disease. The social hour before dinner times forty years equals several barrels of alcohol. Make this diagnosis early for your physician—tell him about your drinking habits.

An overactive thyroid gland (hyperthyroidism) may also produce a tremor. This tremor differs from the tremor of Parkinson's disease in that it is more rapid and has a finer quality. Other symptoms of hyperthyroidism, such as weight loss, heat intolerance and irritability are not found in Parkinson's disease. There should not be a mistaken diagnosis here.

I have mentioned only the more common diseases that produce tremors that might be mistaken for Parkinson's disease. There are some diseases that occur rarely that have symptoms similar to Parkinson's disease, but a discussion of these diseases would not be appropriate in this book.

Rigidity

Rigidity (stiffness) as the initial symptom can be recognized by a variety of changes from your previous state of health. On one occasion I was told by a patient that his golf game was improving. His sole manifestation of Parkinson's disease was rigidity in his left wrist: not breaking the left wrist at impact with a golf stroke facilitates the shot, so his game improved. Those things that we usually perform without thought become an effort when rigidity is present. Buttoning a dress or a shirt becomes difficult and takes more time. Shoelaces can be a real problem. Handwriting becomes smaller and tends to trail off. The normal arm swing when walking is affected. No longer is there a full swing, rather it appears as if you were carrying an object in your hand. I have seen many patients who previously were treated for arthritis or bursitis of the shoulder because they complained of stiffness, shoulder pain and restricted movement. But rigidity due to Parkinson's disease was the real problem. This error in diagnosis is understandable when tremor is absent. Of course, you expect to be less active as you get older. But look carefully at the change from what you could recently do. Perhaps Parkinson's disease, more than age, is the cause. Discuss the stiffness you notice with your doctor, and be specific about the change you see. In all probability, you have been treated in the recent past with some medication that did not improve your condition. Ask your doctor about the possibility of Parkinson's disease.

Bradykinesia

Arising from a chair is an act that takes no thought. Unless bradykinesia is present, that is. Then it becomes a conscious effort and a difficult chore. Spontaneous action such as reaching for an object, inserting a door key, eating and grooming may become deliberate actions, which you may not realize but others will. As time passes, someone may say, "You're performing in slow motion." This should indicate to you that bradykinesia may be present. Your spouse or a friend may notice that you are no longer animated, you seldom smile and you don't blink your eyes very often (due to rigidity and bradykinesia of the facial muscles). When sitting we frequently cross our legs, shift our weight and change our position. Bradykinesia hampers these movements, and you sit relatively motionless. Salivation appears to be increased, but in actuality normal swallowing mechanisms are slowed, hence saliva may dribble. So if you or, more probably, someone close to you, begins to notice that little things are more difficult to do, that you're generally less animated and slower in your movements, you should suspect Parkinson's disease.

Postural Reflexes

Postural reflexes—the reflexes that maintain our bodies upright in space—may be impaired in Parkinson's disease. If these reflexes are impaired, we may fall; frequently the falling is backward. The fall is not preceded by dizziness, lightheadedness or faintness, so there's no warning! This tendency to fall, without provocation, can be the sole manifestation of Parkinson's disease: tremor, rigidity and bradykinesia are absent. Who would think of Parkinson's disease? I would; you should. I was once told by a patient, "Years ago it was 'shake, rattle and roll'; now I shake, rattle and fall backward." This tendency to fall, induced by Parkinson's disease, greatly increases the risk of fracturing a hip, which we all recognize as a bane of the aging population. If you've had a number of unprovoked falls without faintness or dizziness, even if no tremor or stiffness is present, Parkinson's disease should be considered as the probable cause.

Side Effects of Drugs

A recent article in the medical journal *Lancet* stated that a study in Edinburgh found that forty-eight of ninety-five referred cases of Parkinsonism (51%) were drug related. One quarter of the drug-induced Parkinson patients were not able to walk and half needed to be hospitalized." After the offending medicine was discontinued, the Parkinsonian symptoms in two-thirds of these patients disappeared. However, five of the cases that were initially resolved reverted to a Parkinsonian state months later. Prochlorperazine (Compazine) was the most common offending drug in twenty-one cases and in no case did its use seem to be indicated in the first place. Medications other than Compazine that can produce a Parkinsonian-like picture are Thorazine, Stelazine, Mellaril and Haldol.

Far too often patients may not realize what side effects exist. When alarming symptoms develop, they forget to tell their physician what medications they are already taking. If your physician is unaware that you are taking one of the above drugs, he will probably diagnose Parkinson's disease. This can easily happen if you change doctors or move to another city. Worst of all, you may not have been informed of Parkinsonian side effects. Side effects of medications are relatively common and on occasion the side effects are more serious than the problem for which they were prescribed. Ask questions about any side effects of medications that you are taking or that are being prescribed for you.

In treatment of Parkinson's disease there are several medications used: Symmetrel, Sinemet, Parlodel and anticholinergics (Artane, Cogentin, etc.). Your physician will be familiar with all of these medications and will help you discover which is most effective for you. (Also, see chapter 16, Drugs: Side Effects.)

Finally, be aware of yourself. Any change in your gait, a tendency to fall, the appearance of a tremor, unexplained stiffness that decreases your mobility, difficulty with buttons and slowness in your movements should alert you to the possibility of Parkinson's disease. Remember, there are no tests to confirm the diagnosis—just you, your symptoms and your physician. If you become aware of any of these changes, speak to your physician about them.

CHECKLIST

THE symptoms produced by Parkinson's disease have been identified and discussed. This checklist will help you assemble background information for your doctor. You will need to ask your spouse or a friend—anyone who has seen you regularly over the last year—to help answer the questions when another observer is called for.

After going through the checklist, put it aside, then go through it again a month from now and see if there are any changes. Consider it a benchmark against which to measure and evaluate yourself.

1. Have you had difficulty performing these tasks?
    a. tying your shoelaces
    b. buttoning buttons
    c. doing snaps
    d. getting one arm into a dress or a coat
    e. grooming your hair

2. Have you noticed pain and restriction of movement in your shoulder?

3. Compare samples of your handwriting today with something you wrote six months ago. Has your handwriting become smaller and does it trail off?

4. Has anyone observed that your hand shakes when you're sitting or walking?

5. Do you spill food or drink?

6. When you're holding a newspaper does it shake?

7. Are you on target when inserting car or door keys or reaching for an object?

8. Is it more difficult to arise from your easy chair than it was a few months ago?

9. Compare photographs of yourself taken recently with those taken several months ago if possible. Has your posture or facial expression changed?

10. Has anyone remarked that you move in "slow motion"?

11. Do you seem to have more saliva and even dribble at times?

12. Do you feel unsteady when walking? Have you fallen with no warning?

13. When walking, is it necessary to take several small steps to turn a corner?

These questions have been formulated to help you pinpoint the symptoms of Parkinson's disease. If your response to any is yes, you may have accurately identified Parkinson's disease.

14. Alzheimer's Disease and Other Dementias

SHAKESPEARE referred to it in *Hamlet:* "An old man is twice a child." Modern plays have been written about it, and jokes have been told about it. It may be amusing if you're not involved, but catastrophic if you are. Dementias are usually acquired by people over the age of sixty-five, but they may occur earlier. Dementia should be suspected when a person who has otherwise functioned in a normal manner becomes ineffective at his work, cannot manage daily tasks, and has memory lapses. Little changes in one's ability to function often go unnoticed, however. Getting lost in your own neighborhood, forgetting what you ate an hour ago and not recognizing your old friend signal the changes characteristic of early dementia.

Alzheimer's disease is the most frequent cause of dementia. The general symptoms include memory loss, confusion, forgetfulness, misuse of words and difficulty reasoning. These symptoms usually evolve over several months before the problem can be recognized with certainty. A patient with Alzheimer's disease also would exhibit many other manifestations. Both he and his spouse may notice that he has a tendency to misplace or lose articles more frequently. If he is employed, his work performance is not up to par or if retired, his bridge or golf game is no longer sharp. He is not his usual self. Why? Difficult to put your finger on, but something has changed. He lacks interest in the social activities he formerly enjoyed and seems withdrawn even at home. You cannot be sure he'll keep an appointment or balance his checkbook correctly. His ability to recall recent events is impossible and his memory for past events is dimmed. This loss of memory and intellect continues. Eventually he becomes incapacitated physically and needs help with the simplest of daily tasks. The course of this disease can continue from two to twenty years until death occurs. Alzheimer's disease debilitates the patient and emotionally devastates those people around him. The Alzheimer's Disease and Related Disorders Association and support groups offer invaluable help and understanding in this situation.

At any age one may "forget things" for a variety of reasons: not listening, preoccupation, not really caring to listen, misunderstanding, depression.

If you're under fifty, little is thought about your poor memory. If you're over sixty and your memory is fuzzy, you may be at risk for a dementia. The observation of any deficiency (memory loss, confusion, intellectual deterioration) must come from a spouse, friends or companions. The person with early dementia is not aware of it or will deny that any intellectual or memory fault exists.

Now we come to the "just getting older" admonition again. Most of us are not as sharp as we were thirty years ago. Even though we may not be quick in recalling names and events, our memories are still accurate. We may forget something today but remember it tomorrow. Getting older makes us a little slower, but it doesn't mean we have dementia.

The confusion and memory loss resulting from Alzheimer's disease do not differ appreciably from the confusion and memory loss resulting from other causes of dementia. The diagnosis of Alzheimer's disease should be an exclusion diagnosis; that is, all other known causes of dementia, treatable or not treatable, should be ruled out as the cause for the dementia. Once these causes have been excluded, you are left with a presumptive diagnosis of Alzheimer's disease.

It is important that remediable causes of dementia be identified because they *can* be treated. Alzheimer's, at this time, cannot be. What is the physician's approach to the patient with possible Alzheimer's disease? Foremost in his thinking will be the identification of remediable causes of dementia.

The following tests may be ordered in a different sequence by different physicians. The CAT scan of the head will identify the following condition: subdural hematoma, normal pressure hydrocephalus and a brain tumor. These three conditions, presuming that the brain tumor is benign and accessible to the surgeon, are potentially remediable. The CAT scan may also demonstrate a condition called multiple infarctions. This condition is secondary to several strokes and is termed multi-infarct dementia. There is no treatment for this condition. A brainwave tracing, called an electroencephalogram (EEG), may be ordered. This study is frequently abnormal in Alzheimer's disease, subdural hematoma and brain tumor. The EEG will usually be normal in patients who are depressed. Blood studies will be obtained for the following: thyroid function studies to identify hypothyroidism, serum B_{12} levels to identify pernicious anemia, drug screens may be obtained to identify excessive use of tranquilizers, serum electrolytes will identify a low-sodium content in the blood. (If low sodium is present, confusion and bizarre behavior could suggest a dementia.) A lumbar puncture may be performed to obtain a sample of cerebrospinal fluid. This study will identify any acute or chronic infection in the central nervous system.

Neuropsychological testing can help differentiate between an organic dementia, such as Alzheimer's disease, and depression.

This battery of tests seems imposing. In actuality these tests and the results can be obtained in a few days. The tests discussed above identify remediable dementias.

What are the diseases that may be mistaken for Alzheimer's dementia? Remember, these are *treatable* once the diagnosis is established.

Depression

Depression can easily be confused with dementia. We're not talking about someone who's "down" for a few weeks because of personal tragedy. Most of us have had such an experience and with the love and caring of family and friends, accomplish a resolution of the problem and are then able to function. We're talking about those who, in spite of support by family and friends, "can't pull out of it." They become inattentive and are reluctant to communicate. Their behavior is inappropriate, and they become slovenly in their dress and habits. Certainly sounds as if it were a dementia, doesn't it? In a situation such as this, all of the possible causes of dementia should be searched for. If none are identified, a psychiatric evaluation should be obtained before the diagnosis of Alzheimer's disease is considered. Antidepressant medication and counseling will improve many people with depression and make them functional again. Misdiagnosing depression as Alzheimer's disease could leave a potentially treatable disease untreated.

Drugs

I have seen many patients enter my office carrying their "sack." What does the sack contain? Bottles and bottles of medicine! The largest number of different medications I recall one person having was *twelve.* It is unusual for any patient to need that many different medications. The greater the number of medications, the greater the risk of unfavorable side effects and reactions among the medications. There is absolutely no question that as we age, our response to medications changes. That change, on too many occasions, can be disastrous. A five-milligram tablet of Valium might cause slight drowsiness in a thirty-year-old. However, in a sixty-five-year-old the same amount of medication could cause sedation and mild confusion that lasts several hours. The same can be said for other sedatives, tranquilizers and pain medications. Chronic medications, those taken daily for weeks or months, can cause enough confusion that a dementia may be suspected. Many people need a primary physician and specialist for their medical needs. It is not unusual for one physician to prescribe two or three medications, and the other, one or two. The side effects of these medications, individually or collectively, *must* be made known to you. Don't end up being a dementia suspect because of medications. Ask questions regarding possible side effects of all medications you take. Always tell your doctor—every doctor you see—all the medications you take, how much and how often.

Hypothyroidism

Many of us tend to become less active and gain weight as we get older. In spite of this, we're alert and we function in a meaningful fashion. You may notice that your spouse seems to nap more than usual in the daytime and is uninterested in doing things that she previously enjoyed. Within a few weeks, her memory has become poor. The possibility of Alzheimer's disease may occur to you and you see your physician. Results of a blood count and CAT head scan are normal, and the possibility of Alzheimer's disease is considered. Wait: thyroid function studies should be ordered and in this particular situation could confirm the diagnosis of hypothyroidism. These studies are performed on blood that can be drawn right in your doctor's office. The results of the laboratory tests are usually available in three or four days, and medications result in dramatic improvement in four to six weeks. Remember, this is a treatable disease.

Pernicious Anemia

Pernicious anemia is one of the many diseases that in the early stages causes numbness and tingling in the hands and feet. Following the symptoms of numbness and tingling, the gait becomes unsteady. Intertwined with these symptoms are memory loss, irritability and intellectual deterioration. These symptoms evolve over a few months and may easily be mistaken for a dementia. Early diagnosis and treatment will reverse the symptoms of pernicious anemia. The diagnosis is established by a laboratory test that determines the B_{12} level of the blood. Replacement therapy with B_{12} injections should improve the symptoms. This disease masquerades as dementia, such as Alzheimer's disease. The longer the symptoms are present without treatment, the likelihood of successfully reversing them with treatment becomes less and less.

Brain Tumor

I recently saw a seventy-year-old woman who was accompanied by her husband and her daughter.

Their complaint was, "We think she may have Alzheimer's disease." During the preceding six weeks the husband had noticed that his wife seemed more forgetful than usual. She was little concerned with her personal appearance (formerly neat), and she neglected her usual work habits. She had been an excellent bridge player, and her daughter noticed that she was making unpardonable errors. The woman herself had no complaints and felt that her family was overly concerned. Her examination was absolutely normal. The duration of her symptoms was too brief for Alzheimer's disease. The CAT head scan demonstrated a brain tumor in the frontal portion of the brain.

A brain tumor, regardless of whether it is malignant or benign, may thus cause symptoms that suggest a dementia. The course of a brain tumor varies from weeks to years. Slowly growing tumors may produce no symptoms. Symptoms are produced by virtue of the size and location of the tumor. The CAT head scan identifies the tumor in most cases. If it is benign, and the location of the tumor is operable, a cure is possible.

Subdural Hematoma

You slip, fall and strike your head. Dazed momentarily, you go about your business. You might have a headache, you might not; you might mention the incident to your spouse, you might not. If it is mentioned, it is soon forgotten. This is the vague background in which a subdural hematoma develops. A subdural hematoma is usually secondary to head trauma from whatever cause: a fall, auto accident, etc. A subdural hematoma is a blood clot that exerts pressure against the brain. This pressure may produce a variety of symptoms, among which are the symptoms of dementia. These symptoms include headache, forgetfulness, inattention, irritability, drowsiness and confusion. These symptoms can last several weeks or, for that matter, indefinitely or until death. These changes should certainly be recognized by someone as a change from a previous state of health. Obviously, it is important for your physician to be told about any head trauma you may have suffered so that he can consider the possibility of a subdural hematoma. Not all physicians will give consideration to a subdural hematoma, but if you simply mention this possibility, a CAT head scan will be ordered, which should prove the diagnosis. A CAT scan can be performed at a hospital or at a radiology facility. The scan is painless, takes about thirty-five minutes and results are usually available in one day. Subdural hematomas are surgically correctable and what might have been considered a dementia can be cured.

Normal Pressure Hydrocephalus

Normal pressure hydrocephalus occurs frequently enough as an apparent cause of dementia that it deserves consideration. If just one case of normal pressure hydrocephalus is diagnosed after reading this book, it is well worth mentioning it. That will be one less case of "presumed" Alzheimer's disease. The characteristics of normal pressure hydrocephalus are memory loss, confusion and intellectual deterioration in association with an unsteady gait and urinary incontinence. These symptoms may well be present for several months. The symptoms occur because of pressure against brain matter from the enlarged ventricles (the fluid-containing chambers of the brain) that are the result of this condition. Undoubtedly the first diagnosis to be considered will be Alzheimer's disease. One of the initial studies in evaluating Alzheimer's disease is a CAT head scan. The scan is done to see if a tumor or stroke is present, which could explain the symptoms. In addition, the ventricles may be reported as being "normal for age." This means that the ventricles are slightly larger than in a younger person but still within normal limits. If they are greatly increased in size, that information should alert your physician to order confirmatory studies for normal pressure hydrocephalus or refer you to where they can be done. I once saw a sixty-year-old man who "walked funny," according to his wife.

"How long?" I asked.

"About a year now," his wife related.

I asked the man if there were any other problems. His wife responded, "Don't ask him, he hasn't been thinking right for six months."

I then asked, "Has your husband ever urinated in the living room?"

"He's done some strange things," she said, "but he hasn't done that."

His CAT head scan showed huge ventricles. Where is he now? He has consulted a neurosurgeon for confirmation and I hope correction of his normal pressure hydrocephalus.

Subacute Meningitis

Certain fungal infections, notably cryptococcosis, may invade the coverings of the brain. The entry of this fungus is typically through the respiratory tract to the lung and subsequently is blood-borne to the brain. Usually there is headache, but this can be minimal. In addition, there may be memory loss and confusion. This is an unusual cause of apparent dementia, but it is treatable. The diagnosis of these infections is established by examining the spinal fluid and determining the presence of an organism. Spinal fluid is drawn by inserting a needle into the lower back. This can be painful, but the pain lasts only a few minutes. The fluid obtained is examined in the hospital laboratory. Spinal fluid examination is a simple procedure and in my opinion should be included in the diagnostic workup for Alzheimer's disease. Special antibiotics are used in the treatment of this disease and long hospitalization is required. Knowing it is curable, even with a long hospital stay, should make having it more bearable.

Aging does not imply significant intellectual deterioration; we don't "lose it" over sixty-five, we simply do it more slowly. There is no question that the risk of dementia in the aging population is high. The diseases identified here and made more understandable to you may help you establish the diagnosis of a treatable disease that could have been misdiagnosed as Alzheimer's disease. We all hope that future research will identify the cause of Alzheimer's disease, which may then be followed by some effective treatment. Until that time, be aware of treatable causes of dementia.

CHECKLIST

THE behavioral changes of dementia, subtle in the beginning and more apparent and definite with the passage of time, need to be recognized and reported to your doctor. The following will help you.

If you notice that your spouse, friend or companion does any of the following, you may suspect dementia:

1. He has lost interest in current events and neighborhood activities

2. His conversation is no longer spontaneous and often his response is inappropriate and out of context ("Uh-huh, Huh-uh" conversation)

3. When driving home, he takes the wrong turn—he's not sure where he is, even though this is familiar territory

4. He has just hung up the telephone, but he can't remember who he talked with

5. He no longer takes daily walks or other usual forms of exercise and is more content to just sit

6. He does not remember an important date that is meaningful to both of you

7. His personal appearance is neglected

The above checklist identifies changes in behavior relative to normal daily activities. These behavioral changes will suggest a dementia when they are related to your doctor. Since Alzheimer's disease is the leading cause of dementia, this diagnosis will undoubtedly be considered. Now you can suggest to your physician the many other remediable causes of dementia.

15. Amyotrophic Lateral Sclerosis

I don't agree with the philosophy "What you don't know won't hurt you." Amyotrophic lateral sclerosis (ALS) is a bad disease; so is cancer. If a diagnosis of cancer is made, in spite of variations in treatment, the patient knows what to expect. The situation, of course, is different with each person. I believe that most of us need to know the bad news, if that's what it is, and make adjustments relative to the time frame that we are given. Once the diagnosis of amyotrophic lateral sclerosis is established, the average duration of life is about three years. It may vary and be shorter or longer, but seldom does the patient live beyond five years.

What is amyotrophic lateral sclerosis? Also known as Lou Gehrig's disease, it is a disease that affects the motor nerve cells in the brain and spinal cord. Formerly, the most common disease affecting motor nerve cells was polio. Polio is caused by a virus; the cause of amyotrophic lateral sclerosis is unknown at this time.

Symptoms vary from person to person in this disease. In general, weakness is the first symptom. The weakness can involve an arm or a leg; it can involve the facial muscles and the swallowing mechanism. The weakness may first be noticed as an awkwardness or clumsiness in the use of an arm or a leg. Stairs are more difficult to ascend. Opening jars or turning keys becomes more difficult. When eating, you may have a tendency to choke when swallowing. The weakness evolves over a matter of weeks or a few months. These symptoms aren't just suddenly there, as might occur following a stroke. Although muscle cramping is not unusual as we age, it appears more frequently in ALS. The weakness occurs because of muscle wasting, and this becomes apparent with the loss of muscle mass. Wasting of the small muscles in the hand is particularly noticeable. Fasciculations—a quivering or fluttering of muscles beneath the skin—become apparent when wasting occurs. The fasciculations are most apparent after modest exercise, such as walking or going up stairs.

The diagnosis of amyotrophic lateral sclerosis is primarily a clinical diagnosis (a diagnosis established by virtue of the history and physical examination of the patient). The EMG in conjunction with specific neurological findings should establish this diagnosis.

There is a correctable condition that closely resembles amyotrophic lateral sclerosis and it should be searched for before the diagnosis of ALS is made. As we age, degenerative arthritic changes of the vertebrae may occur. The neck or cervical area is particularly susceptible to these changes. If the cervical area is involved, pressure may be exerted against the spinal cord, causing symptoms that may mimic those of ALS. This condition may be diagnosed by an X-ray technique and, if present, may be corrected by a neurosurgical procedure.

Peripheral neuropathies, some of which are associated with muscle wasting and weakness, may also be confused with ALS. Diagnostic tests are available to identify peripheral neuropathies (see chapter 7). Multiple sclerosis on occasion may be mistaken for ALS. This particular differential diagnosis requires the skills of the neurologist and that opinion should be sought. (Also see chapter 14.) Patients who have had polio in their early years may find, twenty or thirty years post-polio, muscle wasting developing in an arm or a leg. This condition is similar to amyotrophic lateral sclerosis, and it seems to run a much longer course than in ALS. If you happen to be a post-polio patient and find a recurrence of muscle wasting, it is important to have a clear-cut diagnosis made. I firmly believe that any condition or disease that can be treated should be ruled out before the diagnosis of an untreatable disease is considered.

The symptoms of amyotrophic lateral sclerosis described here are those found most frequently. Other symptoms of this disease do occur; however, a discussion of them would be beyond the scope of this book.

There is at present time no effective treatment for amyotrophic lateral sclerosis. Medical research is underway, and we hope it will identify the cause of ALS. Only then, I feel, may effective treatment be available.

CHECKLIST

1. Have you decreased the distance of your daily walks because you just can't make it?

2. Have you noticed cramping in your calves during the daytime after modest exercise?

3. Have you noticed twitching of the muscles beneath the skin?

4. Do you choke when eating a simple meal.

5. Have you noticed that the muscles (or the girth) of your arms or legs seem smaller than they were?

16. Drugs: Side Effects

A brief description of neurological symptoms induced by drugs should alert you to the necessity of asking questions of your doctor or pharmacist. Drugs can produce symptoms in some patients that are indistinguishable from a primary disease. In the chapter on Parkinson's disease, mention was made of drug-induced Parkinsonism. Drugs may provoke seizures in certain patients. Peripheral neuropathies may develop with the use of certain drugs in some cases. Apparent dementias have been associated with the use of some drugs. Headaches may be induced in some people by drug use. A situation like that of restless legs (akathisia) has been described previously: facial grimacing and lip smacking may occur with the akathisia; dizziness and loss of equilibrium may occur. Tremors separate and apart from those of Parkinsonism may occur as a side effect of drug use. Blurred vision is not uncommon with the use of particular drugs.

These are but a few of the side effects that may occur in people taking a particular drug. These symptoms fall into the category of an "idiosyncratic" response. The symptoms may occur soon after starting the medication or even weeks later. *Always* inquire about the side reactions of medications you are taking.

The medications listed in this chapter are used in the treatment of the diseases and complaints discussed in this book. (For ease of reference, these diseases and complaints are in alphabetical order.) The *more frequent* side effects of the individual drug will be mentioned. Some side effects are modest, more of a nuisance, and can be tolerated if the medication being used is doing its job. Some side effects are intolerable and demand that the medication being used be abandoned.

It will be apparent as you read about the various side effects that some can be serious. Discontinuing the medication usually relieves the side effect. It is important to know about side effects, not to be alarmed, but to be informed. Remember, if the incidence of serious side effects with a particular drug is high, it will be withdrawn and no longer prescribed.

Sinemet, Parlodel and Symmetrel may cause hypotension and mental confusion. They are frequently used in combination, which may increase the probability of these side effects.

HEADACHE

Pain-relieving medications such as Demerol, Percodan, Talwin, Empirin #3 and #4 and Tylenol #3 and #4 are easy to get hooked on and difficult to discontinue. Stay away from narcotics if at all possible.

Prednisone

Stomach ulceration and/or aggravation of a pre-existing ulcer

Osteoporosis, which could result in vertebral fractures

Muscle weakness

Fluid retention

Increased appetite and weight gain

Inderal (Propranolol)

Slow heart rate

Hypotension: low blood pressure when standing, associated with dizziness and light-headedness

Numbness and/or tingling of hands

Depression

Nausea, vomiting

Gynergen

Nausea, vomiting

Weakness, muscle pain

Numbness and/or tingling of hands

Fiorinal

Drug dependency

Sedation: drowsiness

Dulling of mental alertness

Midrin

Dizziness

Skin rash

MYASTHENIA GRAVIS

Mestinon

Diarrhea, abdominal cramping

Sweating

Skin rash

Muscle cramping and weakness

Prednisone

Stomach ulceration and/or aggravation of a pre-existing ulcer

Osteoporosis, which could result in vertebral fracture

Muscle weakness

Fluid retention

Increased appetite and weight gain

PARKINSON'S DISEASE

Sinemet

Involuntary movements: distract from the tremor of Parkinson's disease

Postural hypotension: low blood pressure when standing, associated with dizziness and light-headedness

Mental changes: confusion, depression

Nausea: "upset stomach"

Parlodel

Postural hypotension: low blood pressure when standing, associated with dizziness and light-headedness

Mental changes: confusion, hallucination

Sedation: drowsiness

Symmetrel

Postural hypotension: low blood pressure when standing, associated with dizziness and light-headedness

Mental changes: confusion, depression, hallucination

Urinary retention

Livedo reticularis: mottling of the skin of the legs that may be associated with swelling of the ankles

Anticholinergics with common side effects:
Artane
Cogentin
Parsidol
Pagitane
Kemadrin

Dry mouth

Blurred vision

Mental changes: confusion, depression, hallucination

Urinary retention

RESTLESS LEGS

Clonopin
Sedation
Drowsiness
Unsteadiness

Confusion

Anemia

SEIZURES

Mysoline

Unsteadiness, dizziness

Nausea, vomiting

Emotional "upset"

Skin rash

Anemia (rarely)

Depakene

Nausea, vomiting

Diarrhea

Sedation

Liver damage; liver function studies should be monitored the first three to six months

Zarontin

Loss of appetite, nausea and vomiting

Low blood count

Sedation: dizziness

Skin rash and hives

Phenobarbital

Dizziness

Skin rash

Nystagmus: jerky eyes

Sedation
Drug dependency

Dilantin
Unsteadiness
Nystagmus: jerky eyes
Slurred speech
Skin rash
Nausea, vomiting
May lower blood count

Tegretol
Can lower blood count to dangerous levels; blood
  count should be checked weekly the first three to
  six months
Dizziness, unsteadiness
Drowsiness
Abnormal liver function studies
Confusion
Blurred vision
Skin rash

Mebaral
Drug dependency
Drowsiness
Confusion
Depression
Skin rash

STROKE

Aspirin

Upset stomach

Aggravation of preexisting ulcer

Ringing in the ears

Skin rash

Persantine

Headache

Dizziness

Nausea

Fainting

Weakness

Anticoagulants (Coumadin is representative)

Spontaneous bleeding: most noticeable in the nose, gums or urinary tract

Skin rash

Fever

Diarrhea

TIC DOULOUREUX (TRIGEMINAL NEURALGIA)

Tegretol

Can lower blood count to dangerous levels; blood count should be checked weekly the first three to six months

Dizziness, unsteadiness

Drowsiness

Abnormal liver function studies

Confusion

Blurred vision

Skin rash

Dilantin

Unsteadiness

Nystagmus: jerky eyes

Slurred speech

Skin rash

Nausea, vomiting

May lower blood count

Afterword

Now that you have read this book, you know about the symptoms that may be identified with various neurological diseases. This knowledge will enable you to help your physician make his diagnosis by telling him exactly what you are feeling. A faster diagnosis means faster relief.

You will notice that I have discussed the various diseases only briefly. Much treatment involves medications, and another book would be necessary to fully discuss their use, side effects, interactions with other drugs and relative costs.

Use the Symptom Index to locate information about the disease that may be responsible for your symptoms. Refer to the Glossary to learn more about medical terms that may be unfamiliar to you; the Glossary also offers cross-references to further information about these terms and what they mean. This will help you to become a better patient.

Before specializing in neurology, I was a general practitioner for many years. I know firsthand about the frustration that comes from having too many patients and not enough time. But I was grateful then, and still am today, to hear a patient's careful description of his symptoms. The listening makes me a better doctor. Help your physician be a better doctor.

Glossary

ABSENCE	The period of time during a seizure in which no conscious awareness is present and a brief arrest of all activity occurs. *See* chapter 11.
AKATHISIA	Involuntary movement of legs induced by drugs. *See* chapters 2 and 8.
AMAUROSIS FUGAX	Transient blindness occurring in one eye. *See* chapter 12.
AMNESIA	Loss of memory for events occurring in a given period of time. *See* chapters 11 and 12.
ANEURYSM	Balloonlike sac on a blood vessel wall. *See* chapter 5.
ANGIOGRAM	Injection of dye into a vessel for visualization of a blockage. *See* chapter 12.
ANTIDEPRESSANT	Medication used to elevate mood and alleviate depression. *See* chapter 14.
APHASIA	Inability to communicate verbally. *See* chapters 11 and 12.
ATAXIA	Unsteadiness of gait. *See* chapter 11.

BENIGN	Does not pose a problem to your general health.
BLEPHAROSPASM	Uncontrolled involuntary closure of the eyes. *See* chapter 8.
BLOOD LIPID LEVELS	A laboratory determination of fat content in the blood. *See* chapter 12.
BRADYKINESIA	Impaired initiation of bodily movements (slow motion). *See* chapter 13.
BUCCAL-LINGUAL	Tongue or cheek/tongue movements. *See* chapter 8.
CARPAL TUNNEL	That area in your wrist through which pass nerves, tendons and blood vessels. *See* chapter 1.
CAT SCAN	Computerized axial tomography, a special X-ray technique used for diagnosis.
CEREBELLUM	That portion of the brain that coordinates deliberate movements and maintains muscle equilibrium.
CLUSTER	Specific type of headache occurring in a cycle or cluster in a given time frame. *See* chapter 5.
COMMON CAROTID ARTERY	That artery pulsating in your neck, blockage of which is the cause of many strokes. *See* chapter 12.
COMPLEX PARTIAL SEIZURE	Formerly referred to as seizures, temporal lobe or psychomotor seizures associated with subjective experiences. *See* chapter 11.

Glossary

DIPLOPIA — Double vision (near or far). *See* chapter 12.

DYSARTHRIA — Slurred, indistinct speech. *See* chapter 12.

ELECTROEN-CEPHALOGRAM (EEG) — A recording of electrical activity of the brain obtained through scalp electrodes. *See* chapter 11.

ELECTRO-MYOGRAM — A recording made by an electromyograph used in the diagnosis of neuromuscular disorders. *See* chapter 9.

EMBOLI — Blood-borne tiny fragments that lodge and obstruct blood flow. *See* chapter 12.

FAMILIAL — Having a tendency to occur in different members of a family greater than chance would allow. *See* chapter 10 and 13.

FASCICULATIONS — Muscular twitching involving contiguous groups of muscle fibers. *See* chapter 15.

FOCAL MOTOR — Seizure activity restricted to one portion of the body: face or arm or leg. *See* chapter 11.

GLOSSO-PHARYNGEAL — Of or relating to both tongue and pharynx. *See* chapter 6.

GUILLAIN-BARRÉ SYNDROME — Rapid ascending loss of strength in arms and legs. *See* chapter 7.

HEMIANOPIA — Loss of the visual field to the right or left, up or down. *See* chapters 5 and 12.

HEMIFACIAL	Involving or affecting one side of the face. *See* chapter 2.
HYPOCHONDRIAC	Person with many symptoms present with no apparent disease being responsible.
HYPOTENSION	A drop in blood pressure that may produce fainting. *See* chapter 4.
IDIOSYNCRATIC	An unusual or particular response to a medication. *See* chapter 16.
IMPOTENCE	Inability to maintain penile erection. *See* chapter 10.
ISCHEMIC	Diminished blood supply due to the obstruction of the inflow of blood. *See* chapter 11 and 12.
MICTURITION	The act of urinating.
MIGRAINE	Paroxysmal headache, usually one-sided, which may be accompanied by neurologic symptoms. *See* chapter 5.
MULTIPLE INFARCATIONS	Several small areas of brain death due to lack of blood supply. *See* chapter 14.
MYOCLONIC JERKS	Sudden, uncontrollable movements of the extremities. *See* chapter 11.
NOCTURNAL	Occurring at night.
NORMAL PRESSURE HYDROCEPHALUS	A condition characterized by dementia, unsteady gait and urinary incontinence. *See* chapter 14.
OPHTHALMOLO-GIST	A physician trained in diseases of the eye.

Glossary

PARESIS — Weakness of a body part due to any cause. *See* chapters 7, 12 and 15.

PARESTHESIA — A distorted sensation not appreciated in the normal sense. *See* chapters 5, 7 and 12.

PAROXYSMAL — Sudden recurring changes from the normal. *See* chapters 5 and 11.

PERIPHERAL NEUROPATHY — A nerve disease commonly signified by sensory or motor symptoms. *See* chapter 7.

POLYMYALGIA RHEUMATICA — Discomfort and pain in the shoulders and thighs. *See* chapter 5.

POSTURAL REFLEX — Righting reflexes that maintain our bodies in space. *See* chapter 13.

PSYCHOMOTOR — Of or relating to complex partial seizures. *See* chapter 11.

PTOSIS — A drooping of the upper eyelid. *See* chapters 9 and 12.

RANDOM — That which happens according to chance.

REMEDIABLE — Functional deficit that can be corrected by treatment or is self-resolving.

RESIDUAL — Permanent symptoms resulting from a disease. *See* chapter 12.

RIGIDITY — Stiffness of muscles and restriction of motion. *See* chapter 13.

SEDIMENTATION RATE — A laboratory test to determine the speed at which red blood cells settle to the bottom of a column of citrated blood. *See* chapter 5.

SENSORIMOTOR — Of, relating to, concerned with or functioning in both sensory and motor aspects of activity. *See* chapter 7.

SEQUELAE — The after effects of a disease. *See* chapter 12.

SUBARACHNOID — One of three coverings of the brain where bleeding may occur. *See* chapter 5.

SUBDURAL HEMATOMA — A blood clot beneath the dural covering of the brain. *See* chapter 14.

SYNCOPE — Brief loss of consciousness with recovery in a short period of time. *See* chapter 4.

SYNDROME — A collection of symptoms relative to one disease.

TARDIVE DYSKINESIA — Drug-induced abnormal involuntary movements. *See* chapter 8.

TEMPORAL ARTERITIS — An inflammatory disease of the arteries of the scalp. *See* chapter 5.

THROMBUS — A clot formed inside the wall of a blood vessel. *See* chapter 12.

THYMOMA — Chest tumor, usually benign, found in association with myasthenia gravis. *See* chapter 9.

Glossary

TRANSIENT ISCHEMIC ATTACK	Neurological signs and symptoms of brief duration due to diminished blood supply. *See* chapter 12.
TREMULOUS	Quivering or shaking which may or may not be apparent.
TRIGEMINAL NEURALGIA	Paroxysms of one-sided facial pain of brief duration. *See* chapter 6.

ABOUT THE MAKING OF THIS BOOK

The text of *Listening to Your Own Body* was set in Baskerville by ComCom, a division of Haddon Craftsmen, Allentown, Pennsylvania. The book was printed and bound by Edwards Brothers, Inc., of Ann Arbor, Michigan. The typography and binding were designed by Tom Suzuki of Falls Church, Virginia.